Sine Syndromes in Rheumatology

Jozef Rovenský • Manfred Herold
Martina Vašáková
Editors

Sine Syndromes in Rheumatology

Springer

Editors
Jozef Rovenský
National Institute of Rheumatic Diseases
Piešťany
Slovakia

Institute of Physiotherapy
Balneology and Therapeutic
Rehabilitation
University of Saint Cyril
and Methodius
Trnava
Piešťany
Slovakia

Manfred Herold
Rheumatology Unit
Department of Internal Medicine IV
Innsbruck Medical University
Innsbruck
Tirol
Austria

Martina Vašáková
Department of Respiratory Medicine
Thomayer University Hospital
with Polyclinic
First Faculty of Medicine
Charles University
Prague
Czech Republic

This title has been previously published in Slovak by Slovak Academic Press 2012

ISBN 978-3-7091-4847-1 ISBN 978-3-7091-1541-1 (eBook)
DOI 10.1007/978-3-7091-1541-1
Springer Wien Heidelberg New York Dordrecht London

Printed on acid-free paper

Springer is part of Springer Science+Business Media (www.springer.com)

Preface

Sine syndromes (SSs) represent a problem in clinical medicine, especially if the diagnosis is not determined by pathognomic findings, e.g., identification of microbial pathogens, sodium-monouratic crystals, etc. SSs are topical especially in diseases defined by diagnostic and/or classification criteria, while in SSs a criterion with nomenclature meaning can also be missed. Early recognition of an SS variant of a considered diagnosis is as urgent as in its completely manifested form, because the prognosis and requirements for the early initiation of efficient therapy are identical. SSs require individual approaches and implementation of the principles of personalized medicine in everyday clinical practice. A patient with an SS has the right to expect the same quality of health care as a patient with a standard manifestation of the same disease. The capability of recognizing an SS does not mean only a challenge for the attending physician, but also a feedback test of his/her expert knowledge.

The diagnosis of inflammatory rheumatic diseases, namely the group of diffuse connective tissue diseases (systemic autoimmune diseases), requires the fulfillment of certain diagnostic and classification criteria, respectively. Widely used scoring systems usually have a reliability given as a percentage and thus the minority of SSs is indirectly taken into account among the whole group of patients. The prerequisite for considering SSs in these diseases at doctors' offices and hospitals is primarily the availability of high-quality information on this topic. A difficult topic is always easier to understand if it is demonstrated in case reports. The monograph of Professor Rovenský et al just uses this effect. A series of case reports describing SSs in inflammatory rheumatic diseases helps to recognize them at an early stage and to initiate early and effective therapy in patients where a schematic approach is insufficient.

The reviewed work is a practical proof of these generalizing postulates. They have a high expert and didactic quality and multi-disciplinary impact, even in acute medicine, as they require early and quick resolution. I am considering publishing the book as an important editor's act that will improve the knowledge of specialists, not only in the field of rheumatology, but also in other subspecialties of internal medicine, pediatrics and laboratory medicine.

Hradec Králové, Czech Republic — Professor Z. Hrnčíř, MD, DSc

Contents

Sine Syndromes in Clinical Manifestation of Dermatomyositis 1
Jozef Rovenský and Martina Vašáková

Clinical and Laboratory Sine Syndromes in Systemic Lupus Erythematosus 11
Jozef Rovenský, Martina Vašáková, Stanislava Blažíčková, and Alena Tuchyňová

Seronegative Antiphospholipid Syndrome 17
Jozef Rovenský

Sine Syndrome in Systemic Sclerosis 23
Jozef Rovenský and Martina Vašáková

From "Sine Syndrome" to Sjögren's Syndrome 31
Dagmar Mozolová, Jozef Rovenský, and Tatiana Sipeki

Undifferentiated Connective Tissue Disease (UCTD) 37
Martina Vašáková

Atypical Forms of Granulomatosis with Polyangiitis (Wegener's) 45
Jozef Rovenský

Granulomatosis with Polyangiitis – Formerly Known as Wegener's Granulomatosis with Limited Manifestation Affecting Only Respiratory System 51
Martina Vašáková

Vasculitis with Thrombosis 59
Manfred Herold

Atypical Course of Rheumatoid Arthritis 65
Jozef Rovenský, Dagmar Mičeková, Zlata Kmečová, Mária Stančíková, Jindřiška Gatterová, Martina Vašáková, Jana Sedláková, Peter Poprac, and Alena Tuchyňová

Absence of Arthritis as a Sign of Sine Syndrome in Still's Disease in Adulthood 75
Jozef Rovenský, Veronika Vargová, Pavol Masaryk, and Elena Košková

Clinical Presentation of Sine Syndrome in Psoriatic Arthritis 81
Jozef Rovenský and Želmíra Macejová

Sine Syndromes in Ankylosing Spondylitis 87
Jiří Štolfa

Tophaceous Gout in the Spine Without Prior Hyperuricemia or Tophi in Other Locations 97
Jozef Rovenský and Jana Sedláková

Clinical and X-ray Findings of Sine Syndrome in Articular Chondrocalcinosis 103
Jozef Rovenský and Mária Krátka

Marfan Syndrome Sine Syndromes 111
Manfred Herold

Index 117

Contributors

Stanislava Blažíčková National Institute of Rheumatic Diseases, Piešťany, Slovakia

Faculty of Health Care and Social Work, Trnava University, Trnava, Slovakia

Jindřiška Gatterová Institute of Rheumatology, Prague, Czech Republic

Manfred Herold, MD, PhD Rheumatology Unit, Department of Internal Medicine VI, Innsbruck Medical University, Innsbruck, Tirol, Austria

Zlata Kmečová Rheumatology Outpatient Department, Roosevelt Hospital, Banská Bystrica, Slovakia

Elena Košková National Institute of Rheumatic Diseases, Piešťany, Slovakia

Mária Krátka National Institute of Rheumatic Diseases, Piešťany, Slovakia

Želmíra Macejová 3rd Department of Internal Medicine, Faculty of Medicine, P. J. Šafárik University and L. Pasteur University Hospital, Košice, Slovakia

Pavol Masaryk National Institute of Rheumatic Diseases, Piešťany, Slovakia

Dagmar Mičeková National Institute of Rheumatic Diseases, Piešťany, Slovakia

Institute of Physiotherapy, Balneology and Therapeutic Rehabilitation, University of Saint Cyril and Methodius, Trnava, Piešťany, Slovakia

Dagmar Mozolová 1st Department of Pediatrics, Faculty of Medicine, Comenius University and University Children's Hospital, Bratislava, Slovakia

Peter Poprac National Institute of Rheumatic Diseases, Piešťany, Slovakia

Institute of Physiotherapy, Balneology and Therapeutic Rehabilitation, University of Saint Cyril and Methodius, Trnava, Piešťany, Slovakia

Jozef Rovenský National Institute of Rheumatic Diseases, Piešťany, Slovakia

Institute of Physiotherapy, Balneology and Therapeutic Rehabilitation, University of Saint Cyril and Methodius, Trnava, Piešťany, Slovakia

Jana Sedláková National Institute of Rheumatic Diseases, Piešťany, Slovakia

Tatiana Sipeki 1st Department of Pediatrics, Faculty of Medicine, Comenius University and University Children's Hospital, Bratislava, Slovakia

Mária Stančíková National Institute of Rheumatic Diseases, Piešťany, Slovakia

Jiří Štolfa Institute of Rheumatology, Prague, Czech Republic

Alena Tuchyňová National Institute of Rheumatic Diseases, Piešťany, Slovakia

Veronika Vargová 1st Department of Pediatrics and Adolescent Medicine, Faculty of Medicine, P. J. Šafárik University and University Children's Hospital, Košice, Slovakia

Martina Vašáková Department of Respiratory Medicine, Thomayer University Hospital with Polyclinic, First Faculty of Medicine, Charles University, Prague, Czech Republic

Sine Syndromes in Clinical Manifestation of Dermatomyositis

Jozef Rovenský and Martina Vašáková

Contents

Case Report 5
Conclusion 9
References 9

Abstract

This paper deals with the problem of sine syndromes in clinical manifestations of dermatomyositis. It presents an overview of the literature of sine syndrome, which is a disease that does not fulfill the diagnostic criteria of dermatomyositis but can have a severe course. In the case report, we describe the development of acute interstitial pneumonia in the course of systemic polymyositis without clinical signs of muscle involvement, but with positivity of anti-Jo 1 antibodies and elevation of myoglobin and troponin. Electromyography did not confirm myositis or a disorder of neuromuscular transmission. The case report points to the need for rheumatologic and immunological examination as well as pneumologic examination of pulmonary interstitial involvement within sine syndrome. It also shows the success of corticosteroid treatment.

J. Rovenský (✉)
National Institute of Rheumatic Diseases, Piešťany. Slovakia

Institute of Physiotherapy, Balneology and Therapeutic Rehabilitation, University of Saint Cyril and Methodius, Trnava, Piešťany, Slovakia
e-mail: jozef.rovensky@nurch.sk

M. Vašáková
Department of Respiratory Medicine, Thomayer University Hospital with Polyclinic, First Faculty of Medicine, Charles University,
Prague, Czech Republic

J. Rovensky et al. (eds.), *Sine Syndromes in Rheumatology*,
DOI 10.1007/978-3-7091-1541-1_1, © Springer-Verlag Wien 2014

The diagnosis of rheumatic diseases is determined according to a set of criteria defined by different groups on the basis of the disease's clinical course and laboratory parameters that enable a nosographic demarcation of a given disease. However, some diseases of diffuse connective tissues that do not fulfill these diagnostic criteria; therefore, it is not possible to determine the diagnosis according to international criteria, even though the course of the disease can be severe.

One such nosological entity is amyopathic dermatomyositis, which has cutaneous signs, but without muscle involvement. Thus, the diagnosis can be anticipated, but it cannot be proven according to diagnostic criteria. Sontheimer [1] published the history of clinical description of dermatomyositis; it is generally accepted that Wagner [2] in 1863 and Unverricht [3] in 1887 described the disease that was called Wagner-Unverricht disease. In 1931, Heinrich Göttron [4] was one of the first physicians who completely described the cutaneous manifestation of dermatomyositis, including atrophic violet papular eruptions, prominently on the dorsal side of MCP joints. However, the relationship between cutaneous and systemic manifestations of dermatomyositis was not described.

During a retrospective analysis of 40 patients with dermatomyositis diagnosed at the Mayo Clinic, O'Leary and Waisman [5] discovered that edema and cutaneous lesions were present in 14 of these patients. They characterized the disease as dermatological involvement at the onset, followed by sub-clinical inflammatory changes of muscles within several weeks or months. In 1942 Harvey Keil [6] gave a detailed description of a cutaneous form of dermatomyositis that was known as "Keil's variant of dermatomyositis." It was an amyopathic form of dermatomyositis that was characterized for many years as a cutaneous form of dermatomyositis with typical cutaneous changes without muscle involvement.

The history of amyopathic dermatomyositis continued with the observation of Pearson [7] in a 6-year-old girl with a florid form of dermatomyositis cutaneous signs, although there were neither clinical signs of muscle involvement nor elevated enzymes for 2 years. Pearson [7] also presented cases of five women who had typical heliotrope rashes with erythematous plaques around the elbow joints, although no muscle damage was found. The disease lasted for 13 years in one patient. Six other patients (four men and two women) had florid rashes; on the other hand, muscle weakness and EMG changes were minimal. Such a variant could be called amyopathic dermatomyositis. Pearson used this term for the first time. However, problems of sine syndrome in amyopathic dermatomyositis continued to be investigated. Krain [8] described cutaneous changes in dermatomyositis without muscle involvement in six patients; however, polymyositis developed later on. The first patient was a 10-year-old girl in whom cutaneous changes preceded muscle disease by 4 months. In the second male patient, cutaneous changes preceded muscle disease by 6 years. In female patients Nos. 3 and 4, cutaneous manifestations preceded muscle disease by 5 years. In male patient No. 5, cutaneous changes worsened and muscle weakness began to be observed after 6 years. In a patient No. 6, pulmonary fibrosis was also confirmed. On the basis of his observations, Krain [8] concluded that failure to recognize dermatomyositis in the absence of muscle weakness – despite the characteristic skin eruptions – results in delayed diagnosis. The disease generally had a worse prognosis if it was resistant to corticosteroid treatment.

In 1977 Bohan et al. [9] published the paper in which they analyzed 153 patients with polymyositis/dermatomyositis; in this group, the authors described three patients who did not develop muscle weakness, although other criteria were fulfilled. On the basis of other findings, it is generally assumed that the interval between cutaneous changes and development of myositic syndrome is less than 2 years, and often less than 6 months.

During the next couple of years other authors pointed out the possibility of sine syndrome in dermatomyositis [10–16] and they suggested that the cutaneous form of dermatomyositis is possible without the presence of the muscular syndrome, while fibrosing alveolitis can occur [10], the therapeutic effect of corticosteroids alone does not necessarily have to appear, and only the combination with antimalarial agents is effective [11]. In subjects younger than 25, cutaneous changes were observed 4 months before the onset of muscular disorder, and in nine patients older than 25, the interval was 8 months. Sontheimer [1] presents his personal experience with amyopathic dermatomyositis in six patients – five adults and one child who unambiguously had cutaneous manifestations of dermatomyositis, but not muscle weakness. There were also no changes in muscle enzyme activity during the first 2 years of the disease. On the basis of clinical experience, it can be stated that if the above-mentioned signs persisted for 6 months or more, but not longer than 24, it was a preliminary form of amyopathic dermatomyositis. In case the signs persisted for more than 24 months, amyopathic dermatomyositis can be reliably confirmed [1, 22]. However, it is necessary to distinguish between amyopathic and hypomyotic dermatomyositis, where sub-clinical manifestation of myopathy are confirmed by paraclinical examinations (EMG, muscle biopsy, MRI) [17] and other techniques including the immunological-disturbed microvasculature of capillary beds from semi-thin slices using *ulex europaeus lectin* [18] and proof of deposits of a C5b9 membrane-attacking complex [19]). Lam et al. [17] presented their own experiences with 40 patients suffering from dermatomyositis, of whom ten were diagnosed with an amyopathic form of dermatomyositis.

Magnetic resonance imaging can play a role in determining the site for biopsy and possibly for repeating it after a certain time as well as in revealing inflammatory changes if amyopathic dermatomyositis is clinically suspected. Sontheimer [1] stated in his paper that a PubMed database contained 49 quotations with the term "amyopathic" in 2001, but only two quotations used the term "dermatomyositis sine myositis" before 1991. The important fact is that amyopathic dermatomyositis does not have to develop only in adults, but also in children. Plamondon and Dent [20] showed that of 27 patients diagnosed with juvenile onset amyopathic dermatomyositis, ten were on systemic therapy and five achieved remission. In other patients who were not treated, remission occurred spontaneously. Filo [19] defines amyopathic dermatomyositis in the case of cutaneous changes preceding myositis by various time intervals. Amyopathic dermatomyositis is thus considered to be a rare but well-defined form of dermatomyositis. It occurs in 2–18 % of patients [7, 9, 21, 22]. Sontheimer [1] defines amyopathic dermatomyositis as confirmed if it persists for at least 2 years with the absence of muscle weakness, without elevated levels of muscle enzymes, and myopathy is not proved even by modern diagnostic procedures. From the immunological point of view, it was observed that in a subgroup of patients with amyopathic dermatomyositis, antipl55 and anti-Se antibodies can be found. However, it is necessary to continue with these investigations [1]. The author mentions in his paper the possibility of analyses of these antibodies in his laboratory in case of suspicion of amyopathic dermatomyositis. It is also necessary to concentrate on amyopathic dermatomyositis from the aspect of organ manifestations, e.g., development of interstitial pulmonary involvement (IPI) [23]. The authors observed its occurrence in ten published cases of dermatomyositis with cutaneous signs without muscle involvement (weakness), while IPI occurred in these patients by less than 6 months after the manifestation of cutaneous signs (the authors used the term "pre-myopathic form of dermatomyositis"). The diseases had a severe course because seven patients died, shortly after the manifestation of cutaneous signs. In a group of 16 patients fulfilling the criteria for amyopathic dermatomyositis, Cao et al. [24] found IPI associated with respiratory problems in three of them; this means that amyopathic dermatomyositis can have fatal complications due to the above-mentioned IPI. From the clinical point of view, patients had a non-productive cough associated with chest X-ray findings and bilateral rales in the basal parts of their lungs. One patient had progressive dyspnea and severe hypoxemia that was resistant to treatment and he died 3 weeks after the manifestation of respiratory symptoms. Pulmonary function tests showed reduced diffuse lung capacity in six patients.

Except for the development of respiratory insufficiency on the basis of IPI in the course of amyopathic dermatomyositis, cancer can also occur within paraneoplastic syndrome. Cao et al. [24] observed the occurrence of pancreatic carcinoma, metastatic adenocarcinoma and nasopharyngeal carcinoma. Another possibility is the development of, for example, a chronic cutaneous form of lupus erythematosus. From the immunological point of view, five of 16 patients with amyopathic dermatomyositis had a granular pattern of ANA; none of them had positive Ro/SS-A, La/SS-B or U1 RNP antibodies for 2 years after the manifestation of cutaneous changes. One patient had positive anti-ds-DNA antibodies. In a patient with chronic cutaneous lupus erythematosus, anti-Ro/SS-A and antiLa/SS-B occurred, but 2 years after the manifestation of cutaneous changes. From the therapeutic point of view, it is initially recommended to administer prednisone (15–40 mg/day). The corticosteroid dose can be reduced in combination with methotrexate or antimalarial drugs. In four patients treated for amyopathic dermatomyositis, malignancy occurred that was resolved by chemotherapy and radiotherapy. Three patients in whom interstitial pulmonary fibrosis (IPF) developed were treated by methylprednisolone (80–120 mg/day) combined with methotrexate. In two patients, cutaneous as well as respiratory problems improved. In one patient, interstitial pulmonary fibrosis had a fatal course despite the treatment. Another possibility is the development of the classic form of dermatomyositis as it was seen in one patient [24]. Pulmonary involvement occurs in PM/DM relatively frequently (5–30 %), usually within the so-called "anti-synthetase syndrome."

The most common type of pulmonary involvement is non-specific interstitial pneumonia, sometimes organizing pneumonia; acute forms can be associated with acute interstitial pneumonia with respiratory distress syndrome and histopathological findings of diffuse alveolar damage. A clinical course of interstitial pulmonary fibrosis can be modified by muscle involvement of respiratory and larynx muscles (recurrent aspirations). IPI in PM/DM can have an acute, subacute or chronic course of interstitium involvement. Acute and subacute courses are defined according to the duration of symptoms, i.e., progressive dyspnea, for less than 3 months. In an acute course, most of the patients are admitted to hospital due to dyspnea; on the other hand, IPI within PM/DM can be asymptomatic. Skin and muscle involvement is usually present; sometimes we can see the amyopathic form of PM/DM; and sometimes even skin involvement can be absent [25–28]. In 90 % of the patients, a chest X-ray does not show any pathologic findings; reticular and reticulonodular changes rarely occur, especially in lower lung fields. With diaphragm involvement, its position is usually elevated and plate atelectases appear in basal parts of the lungs. An HRCT chest scan shows ground glass opacities, reticular structures and peribronchial condensations. Bronchoalveolar lavage fluid contains a higher overall number of cells, and there is a higher percentage of lymphocytes in the differential count, especially in acute and subacute forms. Therapy consists of corticosteroid administration at 0.75–1 mg/kg/day; in acute forms we administer pulse therapy – Solu-Medrol 1,000 mg daily at the beginning of the therapy, usually adding immunosuppressive drugs: cyclophosphamide – pulse regimen with a 500–700 mg monthly dose. Alternatively we can use azathioprine 1–2 mg/kg/day, or cyclosporine 2–3 mg/kg/day. In the case of acute fulminant courses, we can try an intravenous administration of immunoglobulins. Acute IPI in PM/DM can also run a fulminant course and despite the treatment, even half of these patients die due to respiratory failure within 1–2 months (the 5-year survival rate is 35 %). Chronic IPI has an unambiguously better prognosis; the 5-year survival rate is 100 %. With regard to the severity of acute and subacute forms of pulmonary involvement in PM/DM, we have to perform the active screening of IPI. In our case report we demonstrate the occurrence of amyopathic and adermopathic PM/DM with pulmonary involvement as the only clinical manifestation of the disease.

Case Report

We present the case of a patient who was admitted to the Department of Respiratory Medicine, Thomayer University Hospital with Polyclinic, First Faculty of Medicine, Charles University, Prague, Czech Republic. She was transferred from the Department of Internal Medicine of a district hospital with a suspected interstitial pulmonary process, to complete the examinations.

A family history of the patient did not suggest pulmonary or autoimmune diseases. This 69-year-old patient had worked as a shop assistant and was currently retired. She used to breed hens, although at the time she did not have any animals. Three years ago there was mold in the house where she lives, although now the house is free of mold. She denies any allergy to drugs, foods or any inhalation allergens. From the age of 25 she smoked a maximum of ten cigarettes daily, and has not smoked for 25 years. She does not drink alcohol. Gynecologic history: repeated curettages due to polyps, and has never been pregnant. For the last 14 years

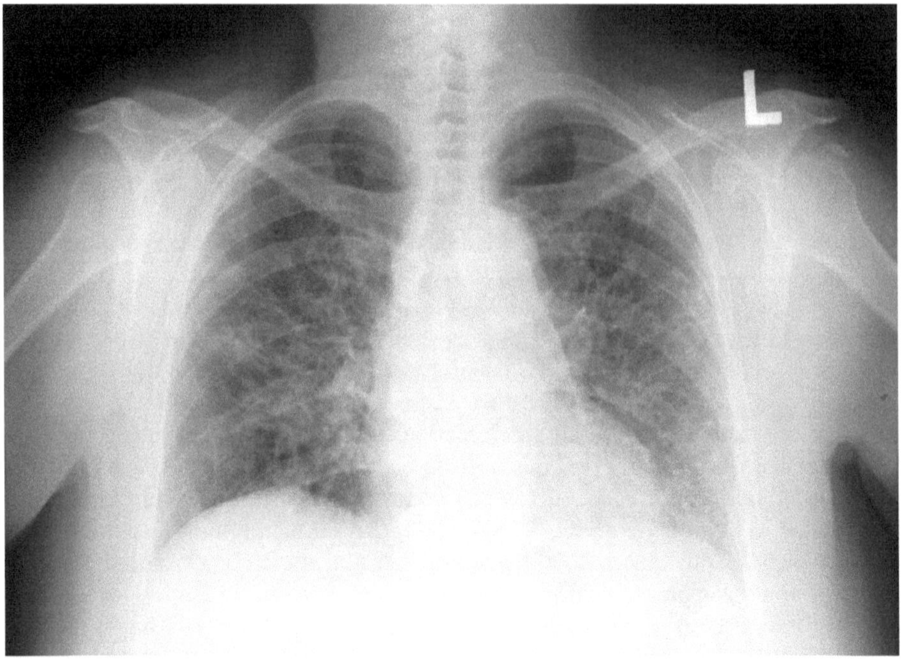

Fig. 1 Chest X-ray showing reticular markings and ground glass opacities in acute interstitial pneumonia

she has been treated for glaucoma and 13 years for hypertension. She has been suffering from chronic venous insufficiency for 10 years. Two years ago she had an injury with shoulder luxation. She suffers from cholecystolithiasis, and an accidentally found cortical cyst of the right kidney, as well as hyperuricemia. She regularly takes the following drugs: Micardis 80 mg 1-0-0, Furon 40 mg 2-0-0, Verospiron 25 mg 1-0-1, Citalec 20 mg 1-0-0 and Lusopress 20 mg 0-0-1.

From April 2010 the patient noticed a non-productive cough and dyspnea on exertion that preceded dyspnea at rest. Rare chest pain was accentuated; she did not tolerate a horizontal position and her legs began to swell. She visited a pneumologist and with regard to radiographic findings was examined because of a suspected intrathoracic sarcoidosis. Due to her worsening condition she had to be hospitalized at the Department of Internal Medicine in Benešov on July 24, 2010. She was admitted with the diagnosis of accelerated hypertension and signs of right-sided decompensated heart failure.

Echocardiography was performed with the finding of pericardial effusion, a dilated left ventricle and signs of pulmonary hypertension. A CT angiography did not confirm a pulmonary embolism; a CT scan showed signs of decompensated heart failure and pulmonary edema, but areas of ground glass opacities did not exclude interstitial pulmonary process (Figs. 1 and 2). On the basis of pneumologic consultation, the patient was admitted to our clinic with this suspicion.

At the time of admission, the patient was afebrile and she did not complain of myalgia or arthralgia. A dry cough, fatigue and dyspnea at rest dominated her

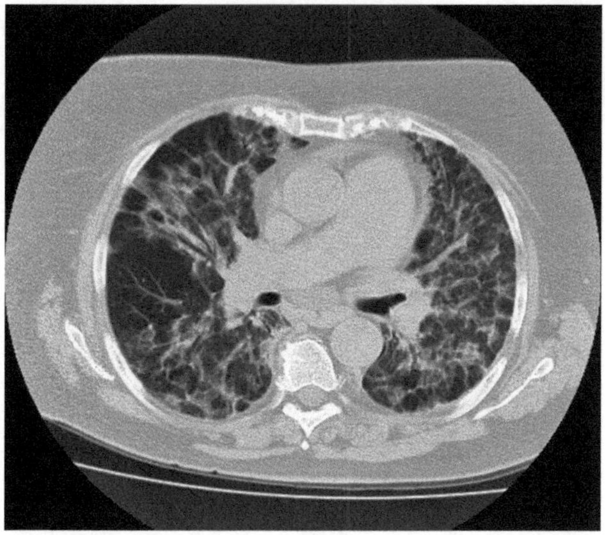

Fig. 2 Chest HRCT scan with the finding of acute interstitial pneumonia before initiation of the treatment

complaints. She lost about 15 kg since April 2010. A physical examination showed obesity and manifest dyspnea at rest; cyanosis and icterus were not present. Rales below both scapulae were present on auscultation, heart rhythm was regular and blood pressure values were normal. Skin was without efflorescence; lower extremities were free of edema. Laboratory results: serum minerals in reference range, initially mildly elevated creatinine and transaminases successively returned to normal, CRP was 23.6 mg/L, NT pro-BNP was 175.6 ng/L. It was interesting that myoglobin was elevated to 71.3 μg/L and troponin was elevated to 0.1 mg/L. Urinalysis showed blood 1+; proteins were negative. a blood count temporarily showed slight leukocytosis (13.7×10^9/L) with relative lymphopenia (7.3 %), RBC count was in the reference range.

An immunological examination was performed, including autoantibodies with isolated positivity of anti-Jo-1 antibodies, and a cytometric examination showed only a clinically insignificant decrease of T-lymphocyte count, CD4 as well as CD8 positive and NK cells. Specific IgGs were examined with regard to the mentioned exposure to mold at home; examined IgG antibodies against molds were not significantly increased. Abdominal ultrasonography revealed hepatic steatosis, multiple cholecystolithiasis and small cysts on the left kidney. A chest X-ray showed diffuse reticular markings with rare nodules. The above-mentioned CT scan was assessed as acute alveolar injury.

A pulmonary function test dated August 5, 2010, confirmed moderately decreased vital capacity and severely decreased diffuse lung capacity (FVC 55 % of predicted value, FEV1 54 % of predicted value, FEV1/FVC 108 %, VC 1.42 (55 %), TLco 14 %, Kco 44 %, RV 91 %, TLC 52 %). Blood gases confirmed severe hypoxemia at rest (pH 7.453, pCO_2 5.04 kPa, pO_2 7.12 kPa, O_2 saturation 89.2 %). A cardiologic examination at the Institute of Clinical and Experimental Medicine (IKEM), with repeated echocardiography, did not demonstrate a cardiac origin of the patient's problems. Despite it, the patient underwent coronarography on August 6, 2010, with

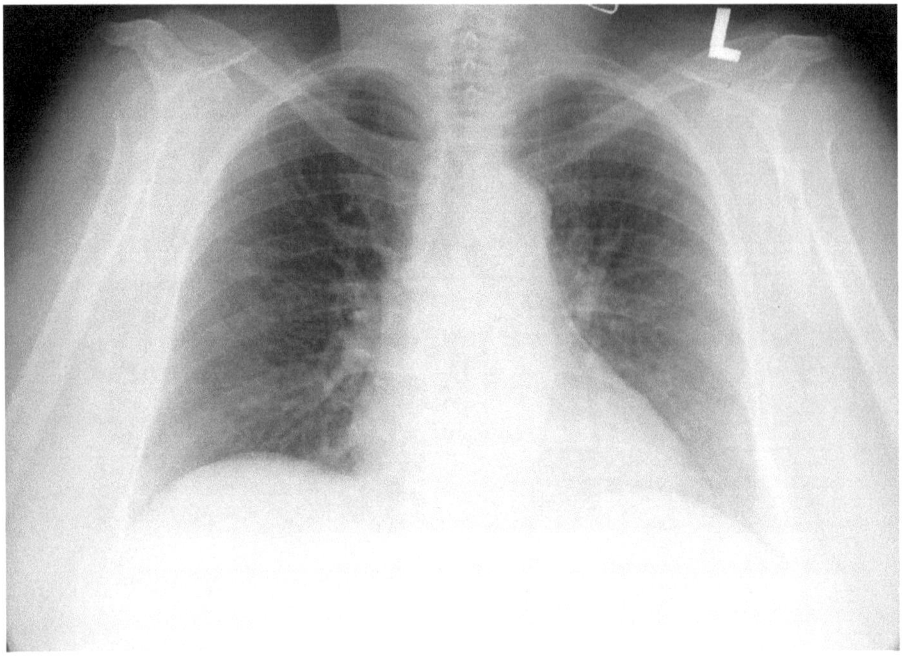

Fig. 3 Chest X-ray with basically complete regression of AIP changes

regard to the elevated troponin and myoglobin levels, with normal findings on coronary arteries. Bronchoalveolar lavage was not performed with respect to the severe hypoxemia at rest.

On the basis of the above-mentioned examinations, we finally diagnosed acute interstitial pneumonia in PM/DM without clinically apparent involvement of muscles and skin. We namely relied on HRCT finding of acute interstitial pneumonia and pulmonary function tests, the positivity of anti-Jo antibodies and elevated myoglobin and troponin levels in normal cardiologic findings. Therefore we initiated corticosteroid therapy – 160 mg of intravenous Solu-Medrol daily. After the initiation of treatment, the patient's condition promptly improved; therefore we began to decrease doses of corticosteroids successively from day 3. A check-up spirometry, dated August 16, 2010, showed a significant improvement of functional parameters (FVC 80 %, FEV1 59 %, FEV1/FVC 81 %, VC 2.06 (80 %), TLco 37 %, Kco 63 %, RV 84 %, TLC 68 %). A check of blood gases confirmed normal respiration (pH 7.395, pCO_2 5.02 kPa, pO_2 9.38 kPa, O_2 saturation 93.7 %), and a chest X-ray (Aug. 16, 2010) showed an apparent regression of reticulonodular markings as well as a smaller heart silhouette, probably due to regression of previously observed pericardial effusion. We definitively concluded the diagnosis as pulmonary involvement of the acute interstitial pneumonia type in the course of systemic polymyositis without clinical symptoms of muscle involvement with positivity of anti-Jo antibodies and elevation of myoglobin and troponin levels.

The patient was discharged to out-patient care with a reduced dosage of corticosteroids (prednisone 20 mg). A follow-up chest X-ray and HRCT scan

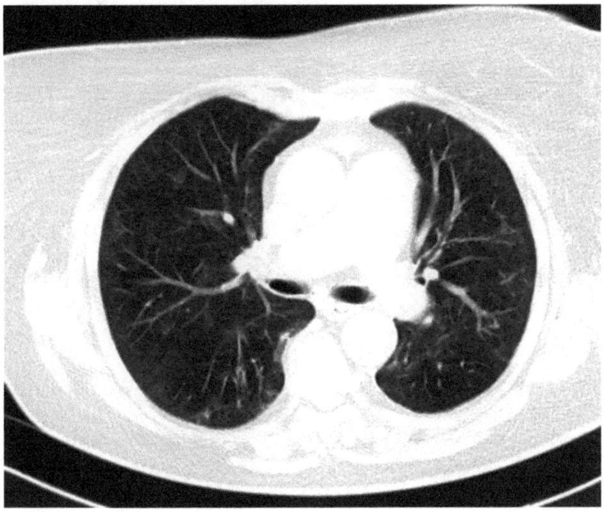

Fig. 4 HRCT scan with nearly complete regression of AIP findings

showed basically normal findings in October 2010 (Figs. 3 and 4). An EMG examination did not confirm myositis or a neuromuscular transmission disorder. This case emphasizes the necessity to perform immunological and probably rheumatological examinations in IPI without clinically apparent connective tissue systemic disease. These can be unapparent forms of systemic diseases that may require modified treatment and follow-up of the patients.

Conclusion

Sine syndromes represent rheumatologic diseases that do not fit diagnostic criteria. In our case it was the development of polymyositis without muscle involvement associated with interstitial lung disease and positivity of anti-Jo antibodies. Early diagnostics and urgent treatment can suppress the symptoms of interstitial lung disease activity within amyopathic and adermopathic PM/DM.

References

1. Sontheimer RD (2002) Would a new name hasten the acceptance of amyopathic dermatomyositis (dermatomyositis sine myositis) as a distinctive subset within the idiopathic inflammatory dermatomyopathies spectrum of clinical illness? J Am Acad Dermatol 46:626–636
2. Wagner E (1863) Fall einer seltenen Muskelkrankheit. Arch Heilkd 4:282
3. Unverricht H (1887) Polymyositis acuta progressiva. Z Klin Med 12:533
4. Göttron H (1931) Haut Veränderungen bei dermatomyositis. In: Lomholt S (ed) VIII. Congress International de Dermatologie. Engelsen and Schröder, Copenhagen
5. O'Leary PA, Waisman M (1940) Dermatomyositis. A study of forty cases. Arch Dermat Syph 41:1001–1019
6. Keil H (1942) Manifestations in the skin and mucous membranes in dermatomyositis with special reference to the differential diagnosis from systemic lupus erythematosus. Ann Intern Med 16:828–871
7. Pearson CM (1979) Chapter 52: Polymyositis and dermatomyositis. In: McCardy DJ (ed) Arthritis (and allied conditions). Lea & Febiger, Philadelphia, pp 742–761

8. Krain L (1975) Dermatomyositis in six patients without initial muscle involvement. Arch Dermatol 111:241–245
9. Bohan A, Peter JB, Bowman RL, Pearson CM (1977) Computer assisted analysis of 153 patients with polymyositis and dermatomyositis. Medicine 56:255–286
10. Fernandes L, Goodwill CJ (1979) Dermatomyositis without apparent myositis, complicated by fibrosing alveolitis. J R Soc Med 72:777–779
11. Braverman I (1981) Connective tissue (rheumatic) diseases. Cutaneous signs of systemic disease. WB Saunders Co, Philadelphia, pp 299–314
12. Woo TY, Callen JP, Voorhees JJ, Bickers DR, Hanno R, Hawkins C (1984) Cutaneous lesions of dermatomyositis are improved by hydroxychloroquine. J Am Acad Dermatol 10:592–600
13. Taieb A, Guichard C, Salamon R, Maleville J (1985) Prognosis in juvenile dermatopolymyositis. A cooperative retrospective study of 70 cases. Pediatr Dermatol 2(4):275–281
14. Gertner E, Urowitz MB (1985) Discordance of skin and muscle involvement in dermatomyositis. Int J Dermatol 24(8):518–519
15. Caro I (1988) A dermatologist's view of polymyositis/dermatomyositis. Clin Dermatol 6:9–14, 47–48
16. Rockerbie NR, Woo TY, Callen JP, Giustina T (1989) Cutaneous changes of dermatomyositis precede muscle weakness. J Am Acad Dermatol 20:629–632
17. Lam WW, Chan H, Chan YL et al (1999) MR imaging in amyopathic dermatomyositis. Acta Radiol 40:69–72
18. Emslie-Smith A, De Visser M, Engel AG (1989) The earliest pathological change in dermatomyositis. Ann Neurol 26:123
19. Filo V (2003) K problematike amyopatickej dermatomyozitídy. Čas Lék Čes 11:142
20. Plamondon S, Dent PB (2000) Juvenile amyopathic dermatomyositis: results of a case finding descriptive survey. J Rheumatol 27:2031–2034
21. Dawkins MA, Jorizzo JL, Walker FO et al (1998) Dermatomyositis: a dermatology-based case series. J Am Acad Dermatol 38:397–404
22. Euwer RL, Sontheimer RD (1991) Amyopathic dermatomyositis (dermatitis sine myositis). Presentation of six new cases and review of the literature. J Am Acad Dermatol 24:959–966
23. Gerami S, Jahromi KT, Ashouri A, Rasoulian G, Heidari A (2005) Sublethal effects of imidacloprid and pymetrozine on the life table parameters of Aphis gossypii Glover (Homopteras Aphididae). Commun Agric Appl Biol Sci 70(4):779–785
24. Cao H, Parikh TN, Zheng J (2009) Amyopathic dermatomyositis or dermatomyositis-like skin diseases: retrospective review of 16 cases with amyopathic dermatomyositis. Clin Rheumatol 28(10):1245–1246
25. Sauty A, Rochat T, Schoch OD, Hamacher J, Kurt AM, Dayer JM, Nicod LP (1997) Pulmonary fibrosis with predominant CD8 lymphocytic alveolitis and anti-Jo-1 antibodies. Eur Respir J 10:2907–2912
26. Marie I, Hachulla E, Cherin P et al (2002) Interstitial lung disease in polymyositis and dermatomyositis. Arthritis Rheum 47:614–622
27. Schwarz MI (1998) The lung in polymyositis. Clin Chest Med 19:701–712
28. Schnabel A, Reuter M, Biederer J et al (2003) Interstitial lung disease in polymyositis and dermatomyositis; clinical course and response to treatment. Semin Arthritis Rheum 32:273–284

Clinical and Laboratory Sine Syndromes in Systemic Lupus Erythematosus

Jozef Rovenský, Martina Vašáková, Stanislava Blažíčková, and Alena Tuchyňová

Contents

Clinical Sine Syndromes in SLE 12
Laboratory Sine Syndromes in SLE 12
Causes of Negative Results of Laboratory Examinations 14
Conclusion 15
References 15

Abstract

Systemic lupus erythematosus (SLE) is a chronic inflammatory disease characterized by varied clinical findings and positivity of autoantibodies. In some patients, the autoantibodies typical for SLE are present, but the clinical symptoms of the disease are absent. Conversely, other patients may have the typical clinical symptoms of SLE, but antinuclear antibodies are absent. Only regular follow-up of individual clinical and immunological signs of the disease enables an early determination of the diagnosis and subsequent initiation of therapy.

J. Rovenský (✉)
National Institute of Rheumatic Diseases, Piešťany, Slovakia

Institute of Physiotherapy, Balneology and Therapeutic Rehabilitation, University of Saint Cyril and Methodius, Trnava, Piešťany, Slovakia
e-mail: jozef.rovensky@nurch.sk

M. Vašáková
Department of Respiratory Medicine, Thomayer University Hospital with Polyclinic, First Faculty of Medicine, Charles University, Prague, Czech Republic

S. Blažíčková
National Institute of Rheumatic Diseases, Nábrežie I. Krasku 4, Piešťany 92112, Slovakia

Faculty of Health Care and Social Work, Trnava University, Trnava, Slovakia

A. Tuchyňová
National Institute of Rheumatic Diseases, Nábrežie I. Krasku 4, Piešťany 92112, Slovakia

J. Rovensky et al. (eds.), *Sine Syndromes in Rheumatology*,
DOI 10.1007/978-3-7091-1541-1_2, © Springer-Verlag Wien 2014

Systemic lupus erythematosus (SLE) is a chronic inflammatory disease characterized by varied clinical findings and positivity of autoantibodies. Disease diagnostics require the presence of at least 4 of 11 diagnostic criteria [1]. Despite this, so-called sine syndromes, either clinical or laboratory, can also occur in this disease.

Clinical Sine Syndromes in SLE

In this case, the positivity of antinuclear antibodies (ANA) or anti-dsDNA antibodies is confirmed by laboratory tests, but clinical symptoms of SLE do not have to be completely manifested to fulfill diagnostic criteria for SLE. In such cases, it is important to decide whether to just observe the patient long-term or to initiate immunosuppressive therapy immediately. As an example, we present the case of a 20-year-old female patient who initially had only minimal pathologic results of urinalysis with elevated activity of urinary enzymes and the presence of ANA antibodies in serum. Other clinical symptoms suggesting SLE were not present. We performed a renal biopsy and the histological examination confirmed the presence of an immune complex deposition in glomeruli. The condition was assessed as SLE and immunosuppressive therapy was initiated, resulting in normal urinalysis findings. During the long-term follow-up of the patient, there were no other clinical signs of SLE and the glomerulonephritis did not recur. Only a low positivity of ANA antibodies persisted in laboratory findings [2].

Another example is of a male patient with a 5-year history of recurrent confirmed erythrocyturia and proteinuria. At age 22, he was admitted to the Clinic of Internal Medicine due to the development of nephrotic syndrome with non-selective proteinuria and hematuria. Other clinical symptoms suggesting SLE were not present. A histological examination revealed lupus glomerulonephritis type IV with active lesions. An autoantibody examination showed only isolated positivity of antinuclear antibodies. On the basis of these findings, the condition was assessed as SLE with nephritis. Pulse therapy with methylprednisolone and cyclophosphamide was initiated, switching to azathioprine later on. The above-mentioned therapy led to remission of the underlying disease. The patient has been followed for 6 years without reactivation of glomerulonephritis or other clinical or immunological signs of SLE.

Laboratory Sine Syndromes in SLE

The other group of sine syndromes is represented by patients with typical clinical symptoms of SLE who repeatedly had negative ANA antibodies. It is seen that about 5 % of the patients with diagnosed SLE have negative ANA antibodies, while they fulfill diagnostic criteria for SLE. ANA-negative SLE has more frequent skin manifestations, photosensitivity, a higher prevalence of anti-Ro antibodies and anti-cytoplasmatic antibodies, and a low occurrence of organ complications such as CNS or renal involvement. The results of the largest published study of patients with ANA-negative SLE [3] confirmed a more frequent occurrence of skin manifestations and relatively lower occurrence of arthritis, serositis, hematologic abnormalities and renal involvement. Kaur [4] described the case of a 13-year-old female patient with a 4-month history of facial erythema and burning skin that was more pronounced after exposure to sunlight, as well as arthralgia, oral ulcerations, hair loss and Raynaud's phenomenon. A skin biopsy was performed, and on the basis of histological examination, the skin affection was verified as lupus. Laboratory parameters showed positivity for the rheumatoid factor and anti-Ro antibodies. ANA and anti-dsDNA antibodies were negative. The occurrence of organ complications in "seronegative" SLE is considered to be less frequent.

Xie [5] described the case of a 30-year-old pregnant patient who developed facial erythema, arthralgia, edema of the lower extremities, positive urinalysis, fever and alopecia in the second month of pregnancy. Seizures became manifested with time. Examined autoantibodies (ANA, anti-dsDNA, anti-Sm, anti-La, rheumatoid factor, aCL, LA and anti-CCP) were negative. Complement components 3 and 4 were slightly lower, proteinuria 2.12 g/24 h was present, Coombs test was positive, small pericardial and pleural effusion was present. A brain MRI scan showed hyperintense focuses of white matter. The condition was assessed as SLE with arthritis, facial erythema, serositis, proteinuria, encephalopathy, lymphopenia and hemolytic anemia. The patient was treated by methylprednisolone and cyclophosphamide. Similarly, a 25-year-old male patient [6] with lupus exanthema, flu-like syndrome, myalgia, muscle weakness, cephalea, vision disturbance, retinal changes and oral ulcerations had histologically verified mild mesangial glomerulonephritis (WHO IIA). Subsequently examined ANA, anti-dsDNA, ENA antibodies and rheumatoid factor were negative. A favorable effect of corticosteroid and immunosuppressive therapy was observed in this patient as well.

Sugisaki [7] published the case of a 28-year-old female patient with fever, facial erythema, neck lymphadenopathy, polyarthritis, progressive proteinuria, mild leukopenia, hypocomplementemia, borderline positivity of anti-dsDNA antibodies, LA positivity and high positivity of anti-P antibodies. ANA antibodies examined by immunofluorescense on Hep2 cells were repeatedly negative.

In another publication, the case of a 28-year-old patient who developed hypertension, edema of the lower extremities and X-ray signs of pulmonary congestion shortly after the fourth delivery, was described. Laboratory parameters showed anemia, elevated BUN and creatinine, leukocyturia, erythrocyturia and proteinuria of 3,000 mg/dL with successive progression to 12 g/24 h. Examined autoantibodies (ANA, dsDNA, ANCA) were negative. A renal biopsy was performed with the histological confirmation of diffuse proliferative glomerulonephritis. Subsequently administered parenteral pulse therapy with methylprednisolone and cyclophosphamide that was switched to oral prednisone led to an improvement in her condition. In the further course of the disease, proteinuria decreased and positivity of ANA antibodies appeared [8]. It can be assumed that the negativity of ANA antibodies was caused by low levels of serum immunoglobulins due to massive proteinuria.

Renal biopsy is important from the diagnostic point of view, especially in those cases where other clinical, biochemical and serologic signs suggesting SLE are absent. In a 16-year-old patient [9] with facial paralysis, rash, alopecia, oral ulcerations, proteinuria of 744 mg/24 h and histologically verified mesangial glomerulonephritis and unspecified leukocytoclastic vasculitis, ANA antibodies were also repeatedly negative. The positivity of anti-Ro antibodies and hypocomplementemia was present. Later on, arthritis, psychosis, pleuritis/pericarditis, lymphopenia and positivity of ANA and anti-dsDNA antibodies developed.

Caltic [10] published the case of a 13-year-old male patient who was admitted to the hospital due to abdominal pain, vomiting and hematemesis. On admission, pretibial edema of the lower extremities with arthritis and petechiae around the ankles, renal involvement with elevated creatinine levels, hypoalbuminemia, hypocomplementemia, proteinuria, hematuria, and serositis (pleural effusion, ascites) were found. Tests for ANA, anti-dsDNA, ANCA and ACLA antibodies were negative. A renal biopsy confirmed diffuse proliferative lupus nephritis. According to clinical presentation, the diagnosis of SLE was made (arthritis, serositis, cutaneous vasculitis, anemia with a positive Coombs test and hypocomplementemia). In spite of the absence of autoantibodies, pulse therapy with methylprednisolone was initiated with a subsequent switch to p.o. prednisone. After temporary improvement, the patient was rehospitalized due to progressive ascites and pleural effusion. A renal biopsy was performed, with lupus nephritis type IV being found. The patient received methylprednisolone pulse therapy i.v. once a month for 6 months and oral cyclophosphamide that was replaced with azathioprin at a later period. A test for autoantibodies was negative.

Cobenas [11] published the case of a 5-month-old girl admitted to the hospital due to weakness, pallor, purpura, thrombocytopenia and anemia with the diagnosis of idiopathic thrombocytopenic purpura; treatment with prednisone was very effective. After stopping the treatment, the disease recurred with a gradual development of hepatosplenomegaly and positivity of the Coombs test. For this, she received methylprednisolone pulses without permanent medication. At the age of 22 months, hypocomplementemia appeared, proteinuria of 300 mg/dL occurred 1 month later, and the nephrotic syndrome with quantitative proteinuria of 4.95 g/L was present at age 26 months. A renal biopsy confirmed membranous glomerulonephritis. ANA, as well as anti-dsDNA antibodies, were repeatedly negative. The condition was diagnosed as ANA-negative SLE with nephritis, hemolytic anemia and thrombocytopenia. The treatment consisted of methylprednisolone and cyclophosphamide pulses with a subsequent switch to azathioprin.

Sharman [12] prefers the term "C1q nephropathy" instead of "seronegative lupus nephritis." In a group of nine patients with a typical histological presentation of lupus nephritis and negative serology, none of them developed other clinical or serological signs of SLE during a 6-year follow-up.

Causes of Negative Results of Laboratory Examinations

Several causes of "seronegative" SLE are presumed. The most frequently used method for the examination of ANA antibodies is the indirect immunofluorescense test. Correct serum dilution is important in this examination [13]. Substrates for

ANA detection also differ from the point of sensitivity. A group of 76 patients with SLE who had negative ANA antibodies examined on rat liver cells had the serum examined by the ELISA test. In all, the originally ANA-negative sera ELISA test revealed elevated levels of anti-Ro/SSA antibodies and nearly half of the patients also had the positivity of anti-La/SSB antibodies. The ELISA test is 10–100 times more sensitive than indirect immunofluorescense. The positivity of anti-Ro/SSA antibodies in gel diffusion is about 68 % and it increases to 92–100 % in the ELISA test [14]. Immunological tests for the detection of anti-dsDNA antibodies differ from the point of specificity and sensitivity. Currently the most frequently used tests are the indirect immunofluorescense test using the *Crithidia luciliae* antigen and the ELISA test with purified dsDNA [15]. Another possible cause is the presence of anti-ribosomal P antibodies (anti-P) that are not detectable by common tests. ANA can also be part of the immune complexes and thus they are not detected in serum. Massive proteinuria can also be the cause of the absence of ANA antibodies due to their excretion in urine [5]. Approximately 10 % of originally ANA-negative cases of SLE become ANA-positive in about 4 years [16].

Conclusion

SLE diagnostics resemble puzzles. A gradual and thorough connection of individual pieces of the puzzle (clinical and laboratory signs that gradually appear) is always necessary, while the presence of nephropathy can be one of the important factors for the diagnosis of seronegative SLE. Therefore it is an important task for general practitioners to monitor a patient with this systemic disease, especially during long-term remission when he/she does not regularly visit a rheumatologist. General practitioners should also perform urinalysis in diagnostically undifferentiated conditions, which can contribute to the earlier detection of patients with lupus nephritis who do not have a typical clinical presentation of SLE.

References

1. Tan EM, Cohen ES, Fries SF et al (1982) The 1982 revised criteria for the classification of systemic lupus erythematosus. Arthritis Rheum 25:1271–1277
2. Žitňan D, Cebecauer L (1973) Systémový lupus erythematosus. Osveta, Martin, p 215
3. Maddison PJ, Provost TT, Reichlin M (1981) Serological findings in patients with "ANA negative" systemic lupus erythematosus. Medicine (Baltimore) 60:87–94
4. Kaur S, Thami GP (2003) Antinuclear antibody-seronegative lupus erythematosus: revisited. Indian J Pediatr 70(2):185–186
5. Xie Q, Liu Y, Yang N et al (2012) Antinuclear antibody-negative systemic lupus erythematosus in a case with pregnancy. Rheumatol Int 32(10):3273–3276
6. Creamer P, Kirwan J (1992) Seronegative systemic lupus erythematosus. Br J Rheumatol 21:619–622
7. Sugisaki K, Takeda I, Kanno T et al (2002) An anti-nuclear antibody-negative patient with systemic lupus erythematosus (SLE) accompanied with anti-ribosomal P antibody (anti- P). Intern Med 41:1047–1051
8. Özdemir FN, Elsurer R, Akcay A et al (2005) Seronegative systemic lupus erythematosus. Lupus 14:629–631

9. Blaustein DA, Blaustein SA (1998) Antinuclear antibody negative systemic lupus erythematosus presenting as bilateral facial paralysis. J Rheumatol 25:798–800
10. Caltik A, Demircin G, Bülbül M et al (2013) An unusual case of ANA negative systemic lupus erythematosus presented with vasculitis, long-standing serositis and full-house nephropathy. Rheumatol Int 33(1):219–222
11. Cobenas CJ, Spizzirri FD (2003) Membranous nephropathy and seronegative systemic lupus erythematosus. Pediatr Nephrol 18:202–203
12. Sharman A, Furness P, Feehally J (2004) Distinguishing Clq nephropathy from lupus nephritis. Nephrol Dial Transplant 19:1420–1426
13. Lukáč J, Cebecauer L (2010) Autoprotilátky pri systémových autoimunitných chorobách. In: Lukáč J et al (eds) Systémové choroby spojivového tkaniva (systémové autoimunitné choroby). PN print, s.r.o, Piešťany, pp 72–82
14. Reichlin M (2000) ANA negative systemic lupus erythematosus sera revisited serologically. Lupus 9:116–119
15. Atta AM, Pereira MM, Santiago M et al (2009) Anti-dsDNA antibodies in Brazilian patients of mainly African descent with systemic lupus erythematosus: lack of association with lupus nephritis. Clin Rheumatol 28:693–697
16. Ahmed AR, Workman S (1983) ANA-negative lupus erythematosus. Clin Exp Dermatol 8: 369–377

Seronegative Antiphospholipid Syndrome

Jozef Rovenský

Contents

Discussion 20
References 20

Abstract

Antiphospholipid syndrome (APS) is an autoimmune disease consisting of clinical symptoms such as arterial and venous thromboses, recurrent spontaneous abortions, and the occasional occurrence of thrombocytopenia.

Antiphospholipid antibodies are present in APS, accompanying the clinical presentation of this disease. We also present the analysis of catastrophic antiphospholipid syndrome (CAPS; also called Asherson's syndrome), which is characterized by acute and multiorgan involvement as a consequence of arterial and venous thromboses. The presence of antiphospholipid antibodies helps the nosographic demarcation of this serious syndrome. As in rheumatoid arthritis and systemic lupus erythematosus, seronegativity also occurs in APS and CAPS. The cause of seronegativity is explained in this chapter. The disease can have a severe course in seronegative APS and CAPS, as discussed here.

Antiphospholipid syndrome (APS) consists of the following clinical signs: arterial and venous thromboses, recurrent abortions, and the occasional occurrence of thrombocytopenia. In addition to these signs, cephalea, migraine, memory loss, an

J. Rovenský
National Institute of Rheumatic Diseases, Piešťany, Slovakia

Institute of Physiotherapy, Balneology and Therapeutic Rehabilitation, University of Saint Cyril and Methodius, Trnava, Piešťany, Slovakia
e-mail: jozef.rovensky@nurch.sk

J. Rovensky et al. (eds.), *Sine Syndromes in Rheumatology*,
DOI 10.1007/978-3-7091-1541-1_3, © Springer-Verlag Wien 2014

atypical form of multiple sclerosis, livedo reticularis, and the involvement of heart valves can occur. (In APS, antiphospholipid antibodies (aPL) are usually present, especially in the IgG class that is associated with the clinical symptoms linked to a thrombosis risk [1].). However, in clinical practice, various discrepancies between the presence of antiphospholipid antibodies and the clinical presentation of the disease in primary as well as in secondary APS occur [2–4, 5, 6, 7]. The number of patients suffering from APS who do not have APS antibodies in serum has recently increased. This is the so-called seronegative APS [7]. Hughes and Khamasta [8] presented cases of seronegative APS. These patients suffered from migraine, stroke, several spontaneous abortions, thrombocytopenia, and livedo reticularis while the tests confirming APS were negative for a long time.

What is seronegative APS and what is its cause? There are three possibilities:

1. The diagnosis can be wrong and the patient suffers from a different coagulopathy.
2. It can be a laboratory problem when conventional tests simply fail because the antibodies are targeted against various phospholipids or protein cofactors.
3. Another possibility is that a previously positive test simply changes to a negative one. The disappearance of aCL antibodies can be the result of consumption in the course of acute thrombosis, more likely developing gradually over an extended time period [5].

Therefore, a different coagulopathy can be present from the clinical syndromes, e.g., that aCL antibodies are still negative in Sneddon's syndrome, which is associated with stroke and livedo reticularis. It is generally known that routine screening tests frequently do not reveal positive results. The antibodies can be targeted against other phospholipids, such as phosphatidylethanolamine, or against the components of protein C pathway or anexin V. The discovery of the beta$_2$-glycoprotein I (beta$_2$GPI) cofactor brings hope that APS screening can be more accurate and that anti-beta$_2$-GPI testing can increase the number of APS cases that were considered to be negative using older testing methods. However, the number of extra seronegative cases was small. The experience of the authors of the paper [8] demonstrates that positivity of beta$_2$GPI antibodies is present in aCL-negative patients. The testing of IgA aCL antibodies did not clearly help increase the number of positive cases. It is possible that previously positive titers of IgA aCL antibodies become negative during an acute thrombotic episode. There are some cases of, for example, pulmonary hypertension, where a history of migraine or recurrent spontaneous abortions can have positive aCL tests in older clinical records.

Just as in seronegative RA or SLE, the problem of seronegative forms can also occur in APS. Sanmarco [9] defined seronegative APS as a typical APS with complete clinical manifestation, but with negative serology. One of the possible explanations is that there can also be APS with complete clinical activity and antiphospholipid antibodies as well as with the presence of clinical activity, but without the APS-antiphospholipid antibodies. The term "seronegative APS" was first used by McCarty [10] in 2000 and later on by Hughes and Khamashta [8]. Sanmarco [9] states that antibodies against phosphatidylethanolamine (APE) can be responsible for the main clinical manifestations of APS. APE can be an independent factor; antibodies are detected only in about 60 % of APS-positive sera in recurrent abortions or thromboses. Therefore it is necessary not to neglect the detection of APE antibodies in seronegative APS [9].

Bertolaccini and Khamashta [11] published the options of seronegative APS when the disease fulfills APS criteria but there is an absence of beta$_2$GPI IgG as well as IgM isotypes. Simultaneously, there is an absence of LA that is recommended by the International Society for Thrombosis and Hemostasis of the working subgroup for detection of lupus anticoagulants – phospholipid-dependent antibodies [2]. This is a small group of patients with classical manifestation of APS, where aCL-antibodies as well as LA are permanently absent. This situation leads to the origin of the concept of seronegative APS. Before the definitive determination of the diagnosis of seronegative APS, it is necessary to continually confirm the absence of the above-mentioned antibodies [11]. Stojanovich et al. [12] highlighted the occurrence of seronegative catastrophic syndrome (CAPS) that is most frequently caused by consumption of aCL-antibodies in acute thrombotic conditions. This belief was also confirmed by previous papers [1, 4, 12, 13, 14].

Our authors highlighted the occurrence of seronegative CAPS presenting with thrombotic microangiopathy that was clinically manifested as severe limb necrosis [10]. CAPS developed after an episode of gastroenteritis; the clinical presentation included kidney and liver damage, and hematologic findings suggested the development of microangiopathic hemolytic anemia. Antiphospholipid antibodies were absent in laboratory findings. Despite comprehensive therapy (plasma exchange, anticoagulant therapy [heparin], parenteral corticosteroid administration, hyperbaric therapy) the patient died from a cerebral hemorrhage.

From the point of seronegativity of aCL antibodies, the authors assume that the decrease or even absence of aCL develops during the formation of thrombi and this can be the cause of aCL negativity in CAPS. Hughes and Khamashta [8] also pointed out this option.

Hrnčiar et al. [15] published the review that documented the lethal case of CAPS in a 51-year-old patient who had CAPS with multiorgan thrombotic-ischemic microvascular damage and with the subsequent failure that resulted in the patient's death. aCL that were negative, probably due to their consumption during the terminal autoimmune storm, were detected in the patient when he was close to death. On the other hand, Sedlák et al. [16] published the case of severe hemolytic-uremic syndrome associated with antiphospholipid antibodies. This clinical and laboratory finding appeared after intestinal infection. It is interesting that large vascular occlusions were not present. The authors believe that it was a variant of APS, the so-called "MAPS."

Miret et al. [17] documented two cases of APS: One was associated with SLE, while APS seronegativity was present; aCL levels were negative during thrombotic events, while aCL antibodies were repeatedly detectable 2–7 months later. Rodriguez-Garcia et al. [7] recently pointed out insignificant differences in the frequency of thrombotic events and gynecologic morbidity in seronegative APS vs. seropositive APS. On the other hand, the incidence of seronegative APS in SLE was lower than seropositive APS in SLE.

Discussion

Patients with typical manifestation of APS in some cases can have seronegativity for aCL and LA, either separately or both. In 1994 Joseph and Scopelitis [18] proposed the term "seronegative APS" and they also described the case of a patient with clinical manifestation of APS with negative aCL. On the other hand, the patient had decreased activity of the fibrinolytic system with elevated I-PAI levels. Before the patient is classified as seronegative, several factors have to be taken into account:

1. There is no absolute coincidence between aCL and LA and in 20–30 % of the patients; one of these parameters does not have to be present.
2. Especially in those situations when there is a low activity of LA, it does not have to be detected in a platelet-free plasma sample. A small number of IgG aCL-negative patients can be positive in other isotypes (IgM and/or IgA) [19].
3. Some patients with seronegativity can occasionally have antibodies against other phospholipids, such as phosphatidylserine, phosphatidylethanolamine, phosphatide acid, and phosphatidylinositol that are not included in common laboratory tests.
4. New results point out the specificity of antiPL for protein-phospholipid complexes rather than for phospholipids alone, and some studies [20] also show that antiCL can recognize the proteins even in the absence of phospholipids. This suggests that some proteins can be the target for aCL, especially those that have a negatively charged surface that allows potential re-configuration of the protein and appearance of new epitopes.
5. A decrease of aCL levels was observed in nephrotic syndrome that contributes to an aCL IgG-level decrease due to loss by urine. Reduced synthesis as well as increased catabolism can also be causes of an aCL IgG- level decrease.
6. A titer of aCL can be considerably reduced in the course of corticosteroid treatment; the correlation between prednisone treatment and their presence was not finally documented [21].
7. Another reason for the absence of aCL or their rapid decrease during thrombotic attacks can be their consumption [13]. Therefore it is necessary from a clinical point of view to continually measure aCL levels after a thrombotic event, probably at 6- to 7-month intervals.
8. It is necessary to take into account factors mentioned in issues 1–7 in order to reliably diagnose seronegative APS [22].

References

1. Asherson RA (2008) The primary, secondary, catastrophic, and seronegative variants of the antiphospholipid syndrome: a personal history long in the making. Semin Thromb Hemost 34(3):227–235
2. Brandt JT, Triplett DA, Alving B et al (1987) Criteria for the diagnosis of lupus anticoagulants: an update. Thromb Haemost 46:1–6

3. Buc M, Rovenský J (2005) Antifosfolipidový syndróm. Rheumatologia 19:111–115
4. Cervera R, Font J, López-Soto A et al (1990) Isotype distribution of anticardiolipin antibodies in systemic lupus erythematosus: prospective analysis of a series of 100 patients. Ann Rheum Dis 49:109–113
5. Lazúrová I, Macejová Z, Tomková S et al (2007) Severe limb necrosis: primary thrombotic microangiopathy or "seronegative" catastrophic antiphospholipid syndrome? A diagnostic dilemma. Clin Rheumatol 26:1737–1740
6. Navarro M, Cervera R, Teixido M et al (1996) Antibodies to endothelial cells and to ß2-glycoprotein I in the antiphospholipid syndrome: prevalence and isotype distribution. Br J Rheumatol 35:523–528
7. Rodriguez-Garcia JL, Bertolaccini ML, Cuadrado MJ et al (2012) Clinical manifestations of antiphospholipid syndrome (APS) with and without antiphospholipid antibodies (the so-called "seronegative APS"). Ann Rheum Dis 71(2):242–244
8. Hughes GRV, Khamashta MA (2003) Seronegative antiphospholipid syndrome. Ann Rheum Dis 62:1127
9. Sanmarco M (2009) Clinical significance of antiphosphatidylethanolamine antibodies in the so-called "seronegative antiphospholipid syndrome". Autoimmun Rev 9:90–92
10. McCarty GA (2000) Seronegative APS (SNAPS) in 53 patients: seroconversion rate at 3,5 years. J Autoimmun 15:0C35
11. Bertolaccini ML, Khamashta MA (2006) Laboratory diagnosis and management challenges in the antiphospholipid syndrome. Lupus 15:172–178
12. Stojanovich L, Marisavljevic D, Rovenský J et al (2009) Clinical and laboratory features of the catastrophic antiphospholipid syndrome. Clin Rev Allergy Immunol 36:74–79
13. Drenkard C, Sánchez-Guerrero J, Alarcon-Segovia D (1989) Fall in antiphospholipid antibody at time of thromboocclusive episodes in systemic lupus erythematosus. J Rheumatol 16:614–617
14. Kitchens CS (1998) Thrombotic storm: when thrombosis begets thrombosis. Am J Med 104:381–385
15. Hrnčiar J, Hrnčiarová M, Rovenský J et al (2009) Katastrofický antifosfolipidový syndróm alebo Ashersonov syndróm. Prehľad problematiky dokumentovaný opisom letálneho prípadu. Rheumatologia 23(4):165–171
16. Sedlák T, Payer J, Horvathová D et al (2008) Severe hemolytic uremia syndrome and antiphospholipid antibodies following bowel infection in the absence of major vascular occlusions: an example of MAPS? Isr Med Assoc J 10:896–898
17. Miret C, Cervera R, Reverter JC et al (1997) Antiphospholipid syndrome without antiphospholipid antibodies at the time of the thrombotic event: transient seronegative antiphospholipid syndrome? Clin Exp Rheumatol 15:541–544
18. Joseph J, Scopelitis E (1994) Case report. Seronegative antiphospholipid syndrome associated with plasminogen activator inhibitor. Lupus 3:201–203
19. Gharavi AE, Harris EN, Asherson RA et al (1987) Anticardiolipin antibodies: isotype distribution and phospholipid specificity. Ann Rheum Dis 46:1–6
20. Roubey RAS (1996) Immunology of the antiphospholipid antibody syndrome. Arthritis Rheum 39(9):1444–1454
21. Silveira LH, Jara LJ, Espinoza LR (1996) Transient disappearance of serum antiphospholipid antibodies can also be due to prednisone therapy. Clin Exp Rheumatol 14:217–226
22. Mujic F, Lloyd M, Cuadrado MJ et al (1995) Prevalence and clinical significance of subungual splinter haemorrhages in patients with the antiphospholipid syndrome. Clin Exp Rheumatol 13:327–331

Sine Syndrome in Systemic Sclerosis

Jozef Rovenský and Martina Vašáková

Contents

Information on ssSSc from Clinical Practice 24
Summary of Presented Cases 25
Original Case Report: A Female Patient with Interstitial Pulmonary Involvement 26
Conclusion 28
References 29

Abstract
The diagnosis of systemic sclerosis without scleroderma requires a careful medical history analysis and search for organ manifestations. Particularly in undifferentiated connective tissue diseases, severe organ changes can occur (heart, lungs, kidneys), but skin involvement does not have to be present or occurs later. The analysis of anti-RNA polymerase III antibodies can help demarcate this rare subgroup of systemic sclerosis.

Systemic sclerosis (SSc) is a rare, chronic, autoimmune disease of unknown etiology. It is characterized by diffuse fibrosis, degenerative changes and vascular abnormalities that affect skin, joints and internal organs (especially the esophagus, gastrointestinal tract, lungs, heart and kidneys). In 1954 Abrams et al. [1], and in

J. Rovenský (✉)
National Institute of Rheumatic Diseases, Nábrežie I. Krasku 4, Piešťany 921 12, Slovakia

Institute of Physiotherapy, Balneology and Therapeutic Rehabilitation, University of Saint Cyril and Methodius, Trnava, Piešťany, Slovakia
e-mail: jozef.rovensky@nurch.sk

M. Vašáková
Department of Respiratory Medicine, Thomayer University Hospital with Polyclinic, First Faculty of Medicine, Charles University, Prague, Czech Republic

J. Rovensky et al. (eds.), *Sine Syndromes in Rheumatology*,
DOI 10.1007/978-3-7091-1541-1_4, © Springer-Verlag Wien 2014

1962 Rodnan and Fennel [2], published the first cases of systemic sclerosis without the presence of scleroderma (ssSSc – systemic sclerosis sine scleroderma). They described four patients: a 51-year-old male and three females, aged 59, 69 and 70, who died of systemic sclerosis with the absence of cutaneous changes. Later on, other cases were described [3–6].

Information on ssSSc from Clinical Practice

Molina et al. [7] described the case of a patient with systemic sclerosis without scleroderma with renal crisis; organ failure was not associated with skin involvement. Symmetrical polyarthritis occurred 6 months later, followed by rapidly progressing renal failure without cutaneous changes. The diagnosis of renal sclerodermic crisis was confirmed histologically. Systemic sclerosis sine scleroderma was suspected and confirmed histologically, with the occurrence of typical cutaneous changes at a later period. Despite aggressive antihypertensive therapy that included ACE inhibitors and hemodialysis, her disease progressed to end-stage renal failure and the patient died. PNAP III antibodies were positive. This case showed scleroderma presentation with polyarthritis similar to rheumatoid arthritis (RA) in 50-year-old woman who subsequently developed renal crisis with malignant hypertension, heart failure and rapid renal failure. A review of the literature suggests that renal crisis in scleroderma can occur in patients without cutaneous changes [2–5, 8]. It is generally known that before ACE inhibitor use, renal crisis could progress to end-stage renal failure, and together with pulmonary and cardiac involvement, it was the most common cause of death in patients with scleroderma [9–11].

Phan et al. [12] described the significance of PNAP III antibodies in the diagnosis of scleroderma in two patients with renal crisis without other clinical symptoms. Both suffered from accelerated hypertension, rapidly progressing renal failure, microangiopathic hemolytic anemia and thrombocytopenia. One of the patients developed finger infarctions at the onset of the disease. However, there was no apparent skin thickening. Capillaroscopy of the nail bed was normal in one of the patients; the other had an incipient blood flow disorder in the capillaries of the nail bed. A renal biopsy showed thrombotic microangiopathy in both cases as well as positivity of PNAP III antibodies. Lomeo et al. [6] presented the case of patients with systemic sclerosis sine scleroderma who had interstitial pulmonary fibrosis as the first manifestation of the disease.

The diagnosis of systemic sclerosis without skin involvement can be very difficult. Okano et al. [13] confirmed positivity of PNAP III antibodies in 57 of 252 patients (22 %) with systemic sclerosis and this test was highly specific. Later on, this autoantibody was detected in 50 of 111 patients with diffuse skin involvement (45 % patients) and in 7 of 114 (6 %) who had limited skin involvement. In a group of 555 patients without skin involvement that were followed up, 48 (9 %) had systemic sclerosis sine scleroderma and 507 (91 %) patients had sclerosis only on the distal parts of the upper and lower extremities (up to the elbow and knee joints respectively) or on the face; it was a limited form of SSc. The average duration of the disease in patients with systemic sclerosis sine scleroderma was 18.6 years, and they did not develop the limited form of systemic sclerosis or any other diffuse connective tissue disease. Clinical and laboratory findings in patients with systemic sclerosis sine scleroderma did not differ in organ involvement, laboratory parameters, presence of autoantibodies or survival rate when compared to patients with the limited form of systemic sclerosis. In the case of pulmonary involvement, the patients with systemic sclerosis without scleroderma unambiguously had an unequivocally higher frequency of dyspnea on mild exertion as well as at rest. There was also a tendency toward reduced CO_2 diffusing capacity below 70 % of the predicted value as well as a higher frequency of primary pulmonary arterial hypertension. The patients with the limited form of systemic sclerosis definitely had more individual skin manifestations, such as digital ulcerations and scars on fingertips, teleangiectasia, swollen fingers, and skin contractures on small hand joints [14].

From the other cases it is necessary to mention the paper of Horn et al. [15], who described the overlap syndrome of systemic sclerosis sine scleroderma and of systemic lupus erythematosus manifested as accelerated hypertension and neuropsychological deficit with epileptic seizures. A renal biopsy showed severe intimal hyperplasia of small renal arteries without the presence of glomerulonephritis. The administration of ACE inhibitors, prednisolone and cyclophosphamide led to complete remission with only minimal brain injury and normal kidney function. PNAP I and III antibodies were present and they remained positive for 2 years. They suggested the relationship to the diagnosis of sclerodermic renal crisis sine scleroderma and the presence of PNAP III antibodies.

Slobodin et al. [16] characterized this nosologic entity – systemic sclerosis sine scleroderma – as a clinically highly variable disease that is usually very benign, but sometimes a rapidly progressive and mutilating form of systemic sclerosis sine scleroderma can also occur.

In 2007 Park et al. [17] presented the case of 59-year-old patient with WPW syndrome and SSc without scleroderma. The clinical and laboratory findings were as follows: Raynaud's phenomenon, positivity of antinuclear and anti-topoisomerase antibodies, development of interstitial pulmonary fibrosis, suspected pulmonary hypertension, and esophagus passage disorder. Skin findings were normal. The medical history contained information on paroxysmal tachycardia together with Raynaud's phenomenon and dyspnea on exertion. An electrophysiological test confirmed the presence of WPW syndrome, and after performing catheter ablation in bypass area the condition improved.

Summary of Presented Cases

On the basis of 28 presented cases up until now, systemic sclerosis sine scleroderma can be diagnosed as undifferentiated connective tissue disease or as overlap syndrome. Such a variant is manifested by ANA positivity, esophagus motility disorder, partial calcinosis, Raynaud's phenomenon, sclerodactyly, and teleangiectasia

(CREST syndrome) without sclerodactyly. It is an incomplete CREST syndrome, often without esophagus motility disorder or without calcinosis. Such patients can often be found in everyday clinical practice; diagnosis of the disease is not difficult and prognosis is good. However, SSc sine scleroderma can also occur in undifferentiated connective tissue disease. Such a form is difficult to diagnose and the patients can develop severe systemic sclerosis with organ involvement before the stiffness and tightness of skin occur. Later development of cutaneous changes occurs in 57 % of the cases, organ manifestations might occur 1 month to 7 years after diagnosis (mean value 2.3 years). It is assumed that systemic sclerosis sine scleroderma can occur without cutaneous changes or sometimes occurs before the manifestation of cutaneous affection.

Original Case Report: A Female Patient with Interstitial Pulmonary Involvement

This case report describes a female patient with interstitial lung disease that was subsequently diagnosed as pulmonary involvement in systemic disease – scleroderma without the symptoms of skin involvement. The 63-year-old patient was admitted to our clinic for the first time in August 2007 with progressive dyspnea that had begun in February 2007. Her family history was negative for pulmonary diseases and immunopathies. The patient had worked as a teacher and currently was retired. She denied exposure to organic and inorganic dust, and she did not breed animals at home. She had never smoked. During the first examination, she denied any disease other than osteoporosis, which was treated with Combikalz and Bonviva. When asked targeted questions, she admitted to pain in the knees and ankles, and she was even examined by a rheumatologist who did not confirm systemic connective tissue disease. She was not allergic to food, drugs, animals, dust or pollen. Since February 2007 she complained of progressive dyspnea on exertion that worsened when walking uphill, but she did not have problems walking on flat ground. She denied coughing, fever, pyrosis, or problems with swallowing. A chest X-ray performed in August 2007 showed visible accentuated bronchovascular markings and basal opacity bilaterally, suggesting a diffuse pulmonary process. An HRCT scan showed fluffy opacities suggesting active alveolitis, small bronchiectasis and mildly enlarged lymphatic nodes in the aortopulmonary window and in the right pulmonary hilus (Fig. 1). On physical examination the patient was slim, without joint deformities, without skin eruptions, without sclerodactyly, without radial fissures around the mouth and stiff subcutaneous tissue. On auscultation, slight crepitations could be heard in the basal parts bilaterally, more on the right side. A lung function test confirmed mild restrictive ventilatory disorder, diffusion was reduced to 59 % of the predicted value, and blood gases showed mild hypoxemia (pO_2 8.552) without hypercapnia. Bronchoscopy with bronchoalveolar lavage was indicated. A cell differential count suggested signs of mixed alveolitis: 47 % of alveolar macrophages, 22 % of lymphocytes, 30 % of neutrophils and 1 % of eosinophils. An immunoregulatory index of CD4+/CD8+ T-lymphocytes was 0.56. Echocardiography did not reveal any pathologic findings, and there were no signs of pulmonary

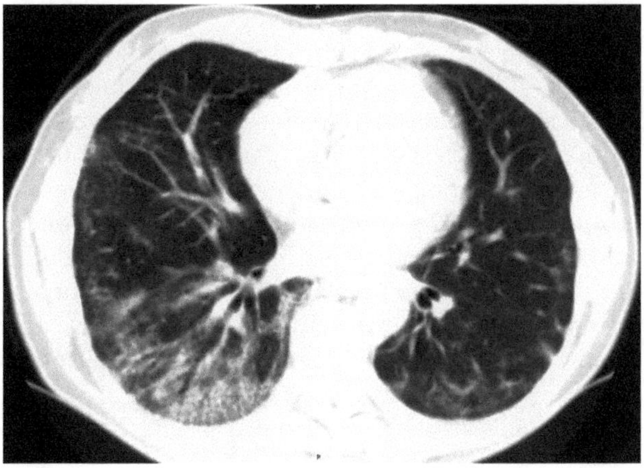

Fig. 1 Chest HRCT scan in the patient with NSIP finding in systemic sclerosis without skin involvement

hypertension. The patient was referred for video-assisted thoracoscopic lung biopsy with taking the samples from the right upper and the right lower pulmonary lobes.

Despite the previous conclusion of a rheumatologist at an out-patient clinic, we took blood for immunological laboratory parameters – cellular and humoral immunity, cytometry and autoantibodies. The patient underwent a lung biopsy without complications and then came to our clinic for a follow-up visit and the results. There was an apparent mild reduction of CD4+ (538 cells/μL) as well as CD8+ lymphocytes (210 cells/μL) in immunological laboratory parameters, without clinical correlation of immunodeficiency: immunoglobulins were within the reference range. The following autoantibodies were positive: ANA 1:1280 with a speckled pattern of fluorescence, RF in IgM class, ENA anti-Jo-1, anti-centromere antibodies and anti-SSA-Ro 52. Other autoantibodies were negative. Histopathological findings from the lung biopsy and biopsy of the mediastinal lymphatic node were: Architecture of lung tissue is preserved, changes in both samples have various focal intensity, but they are temporally homogenous. Alveolar septa are generally widened with various intensity of chronic inflammatory infiltration with the prevailing presence of lymphocytes and plasmatic cells and partially of macrophages. The sections with massive infiltration, namely in bronchioli, also contain an admixture of neutrophil granulocytes. Alveolar lining is preserved, but somewhere it is hyperplastic; alveolar lumen contains, except for desquamated epithelial cells, locations with numerous macrophages, and a small section also contains cholesterol crystals. There is an epithelial bronchialization in a minimal number of alveoli. Fibrosis in septa is mostly mild, but is more severe only in several focuses. There is a dilatation of alveoli filled with edema fluid and rare pneumorrhagia in less affected sections. Pleura has thickened tissue in some of its sections. There are no substantial changes in blood vessels, and there is anthracosis with preserved structure and mild hyperplasia of follicles in the lymphatic node. *Conclusion*: The above-mentioned changes suggest non-specific interstitial pneumonia of the mixed type (NSIP).

After consultation with a rheumatologist in our hospital, we concluded that the diagnosis is systemic scleroderma without skin involvement, with arthritis and lung involvement of the mixed NSIP type. With regard to the presence of anti-Jo-1 autoantibodies, we examined myoglobin that was within the normal values and then began the therapy with methylprednisolone (Medrol), 32 mg daily and azathioprine (Imuran) 50 mg 2 × 1. After 2 months of treatment, the patient came for a visit in a significantly improved condition, without arthralgia and dyspnea. Radiographic examinations showed an apparent regression of interstitial changes and improvement of ventilation to normal, and diffusion remained moderately reduced. The positivity of anti-Jo-1 and anti-centromere antibodies persists; the anti-SSA-Ro 52 autoantibody is already negative. The patient still does not have any skin manifestations of the disease or problems with swallowing or digestion. We can conclude that this case suggests the necessity of a comprehensive approach to a patient with interstitial pulmonary involvement and the importance of searching for even minimal symptoms of systemic disease. In the case of interstitial pulmonary process, we consider lab tests for autoimmunity to be self-evident.

Conclusion

Systemic sclerosis sine scleroderma represents a relatively rare nosologic entity in the field of rheumatology. A special task belongs to general practitioners while monitoring patients with a systemic disease, especially the patients with undifferentiated connective tissue disease. Many patients do not visit rheumatologists regularly (sometimes it is their own fault) if they do not have clinical problems and a clearly determined diagnosis. The rapid (and clinically asymptomatic) progression of organ involvement (kidneys, lungs) can be the reason for a relatively late revelation of organ involvement. These patients are, however, frequently followed by their general practitioners (as a rule, for other diseases), who could check basic laboratory parameters at regular intervals (e.g., urinalysis, creatinine, kidney function tests), which could help the early detection of developing or still asymptomatic organ involvement and thus prevent irreversible damage to these organs. It is necessary to highlight the paper of Mittermayer et al. [18], which drew attention to the significance of PNAP-III antibody positivity that can be associated with the development of renal crisis in scleroderma.

It is also necessary to take into account the development of nephrogenic systemic fibrosis that can be without cutaneous changes, while the exposure to gadolinium-containing contrast agents appears to be a significant risk factor for developing cutaneous changes [19]. No less significant variant of the sine syndrome in SSc with cardiomyopathy and/or interstitial pulmonary involvement is the variant associated with anti-centromere antibodies and CD8+ lymphocytes in bronchoalveolar lavage.

References

1. Abrams HL, Carnes WH, Eaton J (1954) Alimentary tract in disseminated scleroderma with emphasis on small bowel. Arch Intern Med 94:61–81
2. Rodnan GR, Fennel RH (1962) Progressive systemic sclerosis sine scleroderma. JAMA 180:665–670
3. Gouge SF, Wilder K, Welch P et al (1989) Scleroderma renal crisis prior to scleroderma. Am J Kidney Dis 14:236–238
4. Zwettker U, Andrassy K, Walherr R et al (1993) Scleroderma renal crisis as a presenting feature in the absence of skin involvement. Am J Kidney Dis 22:53–56
5. Gonzales EA, Schmulbach E, Bastani B (1994) Scleroderma renal crisis with minimal skin involvement and no serologic evidence of systemic sclerosis. Am J Kidney Dis 23:317–319
6. Lomeo RM, Cornelia RJ, Schabel SI et al (1989) Progressive systemic sclerosis sine scleroderma presenting as pulmonary interstitial fibrosis. Am J Med 87:525–527
7. Molina JF, Anaya JM, Cabrera GE et al (1995) Systemic sclerosis sine scleroderma: an unusual presentation in scleroderma renal crisis. J Rheumatol 22:557–560
8. Canon PJ, Hassar M, Case DB et al (1974) The relationship of hypertension and renal failure in scleroderma (progressive systemic sclerosis) to structural and functional abnormalities of the renal cortical circulation. Medicine (Baltimore) 53:1–46
9. Wefuan J (1993) Pericardial disease in scleroderma: prognosis and clinical associations. Clin Exp Rheumatol 11:582–583
10. Lee P, Langevitz P, Alderice CA et al (1992) Mortality in systemic sclerosis (scleroderma). Q J Med 82:139–148
11. Steen VD, Constantino JP, Shapiro AP et al (1990) Outcome of renal crisis in systemic sclerosis relation to availability of angiotensin converting enzyme (ACE) inhibitors. Ann Intern Med 113:352–357
12. Phan TG, Cass A, Gillin A et al (1999) Anti-RNA polymerase III antibodies in the diagnosis of scleroderma renal crisis sine scleroderma. J Rheumatol 26:2489–2492
13. Okano Y, Steen VD, Medsger TA Jr (1993) Autoantibody reactive with RNA polymerase III in systemic sclerosis. Ann Intern Med 119:1005–1013
14. Poormoghim H, Lucas M, Fertig N et al (2000) Systemic sclerosis sine scleroderma. Arthritis Rheum 43:444–451
15. Horn H, Ottosen P, Junker P (2001) Renal crisis in asclerodermic scleroderma-lupus overlap syndrome. Lupus 10:886–888
16. Slobodin G, Rosner I, Rozenbaum M et al (2002) Systemic sclerosis sine scleroderma: is it always the same disease? Report of three patients and discussion. Rheumatol Int 22(4): 170–172
17. Park YW, Woo H, Yoon HJ et al (2007) Systemic sclerosis sine scleroderma associated with Wolff-Parkinson-White syndrome. Scand J Rheumatol 36:68–70
18. Mittermayer S, Murray B, Hudson M et al (2007) Antibodies to RNA polymerase III in systemic sclerosis detected by ELISA. J Rheumatol 34:1528–1534
19. Todd DJ, Kagan A, Chibnik LB et al (2007) Cutaneous changes of nephrogenic systemic fibrosis: predictor of early mortality and association with gadolinium exposure. Arthritis Rheum 56:3433–3441

From "Sine Syndrome" to Sjögren's Syndrome

Dagmar Mozolová, Jozef Rovenský, and Tatiana Sipeki

Contents

Case Report 32
Discussion 34
References 36

Abstract

Reports on sine syndromes – diseases that have defined clinical syndromes, such as systemic lupus erythematosus, scleroderma, and dermatomyositis with the absence of autoantibodies or, on the contrary, typical immunological features and laboratory tests without clinical symptomatology corresponding to a concrete nosologic entity – have recently appeared in scientific literature on rheumatology.

We present the case of an 11-year-old female patient with a history of Epstein-Barr virus infection with parotitis and lymphadenitis, and who had high humoral activity and high titers of autoantibodies (ANA, ENA, anti-SS-A, and anti-SS-B) during the preliminary examination, without the clinical manifestations that would correspond to lupus erythematosus or Sjögren's syndrome. On admission to the clinic, only lymphadenopathy and mild tumescence of the parotid gland were present. Fatigue, arthralgia, myalgia, gastrointestinal, and ophthalmic signs were repeatedly not found. After 21 months of follow-up, we confirmed a positive Schirmer's test, and a subsequent biopsy of the small salivary glands allowed us to diagnose Sjögren's syndrome.

D. Mozolová • T. Sipeki
1st Department of Pediatrics, Faculty of Medicine,
Comenius University and University Children's Hospital, Bratislava, Slovakia

J. Rovenský (✉)
National Institute of Rheumatic Diseases, Piešťany, Slovakia

Institute of Physiotherapy, Balneology and Therapeutic Rehabilitation,
University of Saint Cyril and Methodius, Trnava, Piešťany, Slovakia
e-mail: jozef.rovensky@nurch.sk

J. Rovensky et al. (eds.), *Sine Syndromes in Rheumatology*,
DOI 10.1007/978-3-7091-1541-1_5, © Springer-Verlag Wien 2014

Case Report

We present the case of an 11-year-old patient. The family history includes celiac disease. The child was her mother's first pregnancy: hypotrophic fetus, birth weight: 2,450 g, height: 47 cm. She was breastfed for 14 months; aleurone was added in the ninth month. She had varicella and laryngitis in the past. Allergic history was negative. Lymphadenopathy was found in February 2010; parotitis was assumed and the patient was treated with cefixime. Laboratory tests showed elevated amylase serum. In April 2010, the patient was prescribed Bronchovaxom at the local hospital, and in May 2010 a significant enlargement of lymphatic nodes and painful tumescence of the right parotid gland appeared. Due to a positive throat swab showing *Streptococcus pneumoniae*, she was given phenoxymethylpenicillin and Wobenzym. Serologic examinations confirmed anti-EBV and anti-CMV antibodies. Isoprinosine was prescribed at a local hospital.

Since that time, the patient had recurrent respiratory infections and was treated with antibiotics again in July and September 2010. Laboratory tests showed a higher erythrocyte sedimentation rate. An ear, nose, and throat examination ruled out focal infection. A cardiologic examination confirmed only a benign murmur. The patient was examined by an oncologist due to enlarged lymphatic nodes in September 2010. Further serology tests ruled out toxocarosis, toxoplasmosis and chlamydial infection. Due to the positivity of antibodies against mycoplasma pneumonia, she was treated with macrolides.

In October 2010 the patient was hospitalized at our clinic without any subjective problems due to many pathologic laboratory findings. On examination she was afebrile, without icterus, but with significantly enlarged lymphatic nodes in the submandibular area and armpits. A systolic murmur was confirmed on auscultation; liver and spleen were not enlarged. Oropharynx examination revealed hypertrophic tonsils without purulent focuses. Arthritis was not present; movement of joints was in the physiologic range.

A blood count showed 5.88 leukocytes on admission with a gradual decrease to 3.9 (SI units), differential count with the predominance of segmented neutrophils, later predominance of non-segmented ones, microcytic anemia, and normal platelet count. Only D-dimer was out of the reference range from hemocoagulation parameters (1882, later 2,777 μg/L).

Biochemical parameters showed slightly elevated serum amylase and phosphorus levels. We were surprised by the high levels of total serum proteins (97 g/L) that successively increased to 101.6 g/L, while the albumin level was within the reference range. CRP as an indicator of acute inflammatory phase was also always within the reference range. A high positivity of the rheumatoid factor was found during the first visit (242.2 IU/mL) and its value was 287.3 IU/mL at the last visit.

Immunoglobulin levels: slightly elevated IgA level and considerably high IgG level of 33.94 g/L that increased to 53.5 g/L at the last visit. Profile of autoantibodies was unexpected: ANA/IF: 4++++, ENA screening: 230 units, SS-A (anti-Ro): 246, SS-B (anti-La): 220, Sm/RNP: 8, Scl: 706, Jo1: 3. ANCA antibodies (p- and c-subtype) as well as ACLA antibodies were negative during the entire follow-up.

Table 1 Autoantibody profile in longitudinal follow-up of our patient

Date	ANA/IF (negative to ++++)	ENA (N: 0–9 U/ml)	Ro (N: 0–9 U/mL)	La (N: 0–9 U/mL)	Sm/RNP (N: 0–9 U/mL)	Sm (N: 0–9 U/mL)
October 2010	Positive ++++HG	230	246	220	8	4
November 2010 NIRD	Positive +++G	Positive	300	Negative	Negative	Negative
March 2011	Positive ++++HG	66	More than 200	47	38	30
July 2011	Positive ++++HG	59	60	8	5	4
October 2011	Positive	77	60	27	12	10

Explanatory notes: *ANA/IF* antinuclear antibodies detected by screening method, *ENA* extractable nuclear antigen detected by screening method, *Ro* anti-Ro (SS-A) autoantibodies, *La* anti-La (SS-B) antibodies, *Sm/RNP* anti-Sm/RNP autoantibodies, *Sm* Sm autoantibody, *HG* homogenous granular type of immunofluorescence, *G* granular type of immunofluorescence

Table 2 Selected laboratory parameters in longitudinal follow-up of our patient

Date	ESR	WBC	CRP	RF	TP	IgG	CIC
October 2010	91/130[a]	5.88 3.9[a]	Negative	242[a]	97[a] 101.6[a]	33.94[a]	198[a]
March 2011	101/129[a]	4.88	–	287.3[a]	–	53.5[a]	185[a]
July 2011	110/134[a]	4.5	Negative	271.5[a]	98.8[a]	54.5[a]	146[a]
October 2011	80/122[a]	4.29	Negative	258.8[a]	105.1[a]	58.4[a]	147[a]

Explanatory notes: *ESR* erythrocyte sedimentation rate, *WBC* white blood cells, *CRP* C-reactive protein, *RF* rheumatoid factor, *TP* total serum proteins, *IgG* immunoglobulin G, *CIC* circulating immune complexes

[a]Values out of reference range

Therefore we repeated the testing for ANA antibodies in National Institute of Rheumatic Diseases Piešťany. Only the SS-B was negative when compared to our results; other findings were the same. Results of autoantibody tests as well as selected laboratory parameters in longitudinal follow-up are shown in Tables 1 and 2.

Other examinations: urinalysis was negative, Bence-Jones protein was also negative, thyroid hormones were within the reference range. Brucellosis, tularemia and listeriosis were ruled out as a possible etiology of lymphadenopathy, Yersinia serological tests were negative. A Mantoux II test was negative.

Oncomarkers: slightly elevated tymidinkinase, CEA (embryonal carcinoma) and NSE (neuron specific enolase) were negative.

We repeated tests that had already been done at the out-patient clinic – the ENT examination recommended re-adenotomy; the ophthalmology examination did not confirm uveitis; and Schirmer's test was repeatedly not possible to assess due to poor cooperation on the part of the patient. A chest X-ray did not show any focal changes. Abdominal ultrasonography did not reveal pathologic changes, but small mesenterial lymphatic nodes were found in the paraumbilical area.

Neck ultrasonography documented bilateral lymphadenopathy, parotid and submandibular glands probably modified by inflammation. An infectologic consultation confirmed EBV and CMV infections in the past.

Bone marrow and trepanobiopsy examinations were confronted at two different institutions, while the immunophenotypization of bone marrow did not find pathologic phenotypes or atypical changes in the B and T line. The impression from extirpated lymphatic nodes also did not confirm a malignancy, and a lymphoproliferative disease was also not confirmed.

We continued in our search; abdominal sonography did not confirm chronic inflammatory changes in the bowels.

The girl was discharged to out-patient care without therapy. During the last visit, at the beginning of March 2011, she did not complain of fatigue, nor have fever or joint problems. She did not lose hair, denied dry eyes and mucous membranes. On examination she was paler, but without significantly enlarged lymphatic nodes; other findings were physiological. The positivity of ANA and ENA, high rheumatoid factor, high ESR with negative CRP, and enormously high levels of total protein and IgG persisted.

We continued to observe the child with completely developed laboratory features suggesting Sjögren's syndrome with discrete involvement of salivary glands.

In the ophthalmology clinic where the child was repeatedly examined, positivity of Schirmer's test was confirmed but she did not require artificial tears during common activities and she did not complain of burning eyes; even repeated inquiries that would suggest dryness of mucous membranes did not confirm such manifestations.

After another interview with the parents, we obtained consent to perform a biopsy of small salivary glands from the lower lip. Microscopic findings were as follows: representative samples containing small salivary glands with the finding of periductal intralobular lymphoid infiltrates, focus score: 3 in 4 mm^2. Conclusion: histomorphological findings support the clinical diagnosis of Sjögren's syndrome.

The child was discharged with antimalarial drugs that her mother spontaneously discontinued after 1 week. In the period between her hospital discharge and her last visit, she overcame herpes zoster that was localized in the lumbar, os ilium and mons pubis areas in an uncomplicated course.

Discussion

Sjögren's syndrome ("sicca syndrome") is a chronic autoimmune disease that is dominated by xerostomia and xerophtalmia – involvement of exocrine glands caused by their plasmocellular infiltration. Sjögren's syndrome can occur as a primary nosologic entity, or it is a diseases accompanying rheumatoid arthritis or systemic lupus erythematosus when it is considered to be secondary [3, 5, 6, 8].

Sjögren's syndrome rarely occurs in children. Its development is slow and it can be nearly completely asymptomatic for a long time. The examination of autoantibodies that are not conventionally examined in common infections can reveal the initial stages of the disease, as was the case with our patient.

References to so-called "sine syndromes," which have a typical clinical manifestation, currently appear in the literature, but laboratory and immunological features are absent or, on the contrary, laboratory and immunological features are present but the disease is clinically "silent." Such "sine syndromes" are most frequently mentioned in association with systemic lupus erythematosus or systemic sclerosis [7, 9]. A statistical comparison of the association of organ manifestations in systemic lupus erythematosus with ANA negativity has shown that such an ANA-negative SLE has more frequent cutaneous changes, photosensitivity and more frequently positive anti-Ro or anti-La antibodies, while serious organ involvement (kidneys, central nervous system) is less frequent. Several authors have presented individual cases of patients that could be included among the so-called "sine syndromes," but in some cases there is discrete clinical symptomatology or simultaneous presence of anti-Ro or anti-La antibodies, or even borderline positivity of anti-dsDNA antibodies. It is most probably caused by fluctuating immunological activity in a certain time interval [3, 8, 10].

From this point of view we can consider our patient as having developed Sjögren's syndrome with an EBV infection as the trigger, with completely developed laboratory and immunological profile without clinical symptomatology. The first classical criteria – ophthalmic signs (positive Schirmer's test) and positive biopsy of small salivary glands – appeared nearly 2 years after the onset of the disease.

Diagnostic criteria for Sjögren's syndrome have been developed, supplemented and extended until today; therefore we can encounter with Californian (known as Fox) criteria, Copenhagen and Japanese criteria in the literature. The most recent criteria are those established by the American-European Consensus group [1, 2, 4, 6, 11].

It is probably just a matter of time until there will be similar publications with relation to other systemic connective tissue diseases that can run a nearly asymptomatic course for a longer period of time. Therefore it is important to carry out longitudinal follow-ups of the patients with incomplete clinical or laboratory features that can help in differential diagnostic processes. Due to lymphadenopathy, high ESR, and leukopenia in our patient, we also had to rule out lymphoproliferative disease of a malignant character, because sources mention the high risk of developing malignancies with Sjögren's syndrome [3, 6, 8].

In some cases, diagnostics of these "sine" syndromes is very difficult, because for a definite diagnosis it is necessary to meet principal diagnostic criteria (or a certain number of them) that are generally accepted on the basis of results of multicenter studies and observations. Testing for ANA autoantibodies (anti-Ro – SS-A or anti-La – SS-B) has the same importance as well as positive histological findings in bioptic material from salivary glands [1–3, 10, 11]. Various diagnostic modalities – sialography, magnetic resonance imaging, Schirmer's test, etc. – supplement the diagnostic "mosaic" of Sjögren's syndrome. The presence of anti-Ro antibodies is important because of the possible development of neonatal lupus with complete heart block and the urgent need to implant a pacemaker. It means that the danger of positive anti-Ro antibodies because of the development of neonatal lupus with complete heart block requires the follow-up of women of child-bearing potential in case of anticipated pregnancy.

This autoimmune disease belongs to the group of systemic connective tissue diseases; therefore it does not differ in multi-systemic involvement including episodic arthritis. Involvement of individual organs can be observed only after a long-term follow-up of patients with this disease, since, as we mentioned before, the manifestation of individual signs occurs at different times in different patients. This implies that it is necessary to treat patients early to prevent or postpone organ involvement.

References

1. Fox RI, Robinson CA, Curd JG, Kozin F, Howell FV (1986) Sjögren's syndrome proposed criteria for classification. Arthritis Rheum 29:577–586
2. Homma M, Tojo T, Akizuki M, Yagamata H (1986) Criteria for Sjögren's syndrome in Japan. Scand J Rheumatol Suppl 61:26–27
3. Lukáč J, Lukáčová O (2010) Sjögrenov syndróm. In: Lukáč J et al (eds) Systémové choroby spojivového tkaniva (systémové autoimunitné choroby). PN Print, s.r.o, Piešťany, pp 219–226
4. Manthrope R, Oxholm P, Prause JU, Schiödt M (1986) The Copenhagen criteria for Sjögren's syndrome. Scand J Rheumatol Suppl 61:19–21
5. Mičeková D, Rybár I, Mlynáriková V, Rovenský J (2008) Sjögrenov syndróm – priebeh, diagnostika. Via Practica 5:80–84
6. Moutsopoulos HM, Tzioufas AG (1994) Sjögren's syndrome. In: Klippel JH, Dieppe PA (eds) Rheumatology. Mosby, London, p 1760, 6/27.1–6/27.12
7. Ozdemir FN, Elsurer R, Akcay A et al (2005) Seronegative systemic lupus erythematosus. Lupus 14:629–631
8. Rovenský J, Cebecauer L, Lukáč J (1998) Klinický význam autoprotilátok pri systémových chorobách spojivového tkaniva. In: Rovenský J et al (eds) Reumatológia v teórii a praxi. V. Osveta, Martin, pp 235–262
9. Rovenský J, Vašáková M (2010) Sine syndróm pri systémovej skleróze. Via Practica 7(6): 262–265
10. Vencovský J (2000) Antinukleárne protilátky. In: Rovenský J, Pavelka K et al (eds) Klinická reumatológia. Osveta, Martin, pp 115–126
11. Vitali C, Bombardieri S, Jonsson R, Moutsopoulos HM, Alexander EL, Carsons SE, Daniels TE, Fox PC, Fox RI, Kassan SS, Pillemer SR, Talai N, Weisman MH, The European Study Group on Classification Criteria for Sjögren's Syndrome (2002) Classification criteria for Sjögren's syndrome: a revised version of the European criteria proposed by the American-European consensus group. Ann Rheum Dis 61:554–558

Undifferentiated Connective Tissue Disease (UCTD)

Martina Vašáková

Contents

Introduction 38
Diagnosis 38
Criteria for Diagnosis 38
Radiological Findings 38
Cytologic and Histopathologic Findings 39
Case Report of Idiopathic Pulmonary Fibrosis That Was Not Idiopathic 39
Our Examination 40
Diagnosis and Treatment 42
Conclusion 43
Bibliography 43

Abstract

UCTD presents as a symptom or a set of symptoms suggesting systemic connective tissue disease (SCTD) occurring together with the positivity of autoantibodies, lasting longer than 12 months. Pulmonary involvement mostly with the picture of non-specific interstitial pneumonia (NSIP) is the part of UCTD very frequently. Criteria for the diagnosis of IIP within UCTD are not strict: at least one symptom of SCTD, at least one sign of a systemic inflammatory process, predominance of hazy opacities on chest HRCT scan, and histopathological proof of NSIP. Fifty percent of patients with NSIP fulfill these criteria when compared to only 5 % of patients with a confirmed diagnosis of idiopathic pulmonary fibrosis (IPF). In our case report we are describing the patient fulfilling these diagnostic criteria but having the less frequent histopathologic pattern of UIP.

M. Vašáková
Department of Respiratory Medicine, Thomayer University Hospital with Polyclinic, First Faculty of Medicine, Charles University, Prague, Czech Republic
e-mail: martina.vasakova@ftn.cz

J. Rovensky et al. (eds.), *Sine Syndromes in Rheumatology*,
DOI 10.1007/978-3-7091-1541-1_6, © Springer-Verlag Wien 2014

Introduction

UCTD presents as a symptom or a set of symptoms suggesting systemic connective tissue disease (SCTD) occurring together with the positivity of autoantibodies, lasting longer than 12 months. It is not possible to precisely assign the disease to any SCTD, and only in a small number of patients does a really specific SCTD develop over time. Pulmonary involvement with the picture of non-specific interstitial pneumonia (NSIP) is the part of UCTD very frequently. Some authors speculate that many cases of so-called idiopathic NSIP are basically part of UCTD, and there are also hypotheses that the so-called idiopathic interstitial pneumonia (especially NSIP, and to a lesser extent, idiopathic pulmonary fibrosis type usual interstitial pneumonia – IPF-UIP), can be the masked forms of SCTD. Interstitial pneumonia (NSIP as well as IPF) within UCTD differs from idiopathic interstitial pneumonia (IIP) in usually having a better prognosis.

Diagnosis

Criteria for Diagnosis

Criteria for the diagnosis of IIP within UCTD are not strict; the most commonly used come from Kinder et al.: female, at least one symptom of SCTD (Raynaud's phenomenon, arthralgia, joint edema, photosensitivity, weight loss, morning stiffness, sicca syndrome, dysphagia, fever, gastroesophageal reflux, skin changes, oral ulcerations, non-androgenic alopecia, proximal muscle weakness), at least one sign of a systemic inflammatory process (positivity of ANA, RF, anti Scl-70, anti SS-A or SS-B, anti Jo-1, doubled ESR, elevated CRP), predominance of hazy opacities on chest HRCT scan, and histopathological proof of NSIP. Fifty percent of patients with NSIP fulfill these criteria when compared to only 5 % of patients with a confirmed diagnosis of idiopathic pulmonary fibrosis (IPF).

Radiological Findings

NSIP. *Chest X-ray*: Patchy and focal opacities with haziness of lung parenchyma, or even reticular changes, predominate in middle and lower lung fields. *Chest HRCT scan*: Bilateral symmetrical ground glass opacities. Reticular changes that represent fibrosis appear with disease progress and coarse reticulation with wider bands prevails in final stages. Traction bronchiectasis sometimes appears; honeycomb lung is exceptional. Wider irregular linear opacities are quite frequent in later stages.

IPF. *Chest X-ray*: Fine bilateral reticular changes can be found in early stages, especially in lower lung fields and in axillary parts of the lungs. The patient can be asymptomatic in this phase, but there are also cases where a chest X-ray can be normal even if the respiratory problems are already present. Reticular and even reticulonodular changes with cysts of 2–20 mm are accentuated with the progression of the disease and a picture of honeycomb lung is present. Reduced lung volume with higher position of the diaphragm occurs simultaneously. Slight enlargement of intrathoracic lymphatic nodes is present as well. Pleural effusion is a sporadic finding. *HRCT*: IPF is characterized by the picture of usual interstitial pneumonia (UIP) that results in subpleural and basal reticular changes with thick-walled cysts of various sizes and honeycomb lung that is present in more than 90 % of the patients. Traction bronchiectasis or bronchiolectasis are common findings. Traction bronchiectasis is one of the principal conditions to set the diagnosis of IPF. There is fibrous tissue among the cysts, and lung volume is reduced due to retraction. Distortion of lung architecture is usually present.

Cytologic and Histopathologic Findings

Bronchoalveolar lavage (*BAL*). More pronounced lymphocytosis is found in BAL fluid in IPF and NSIP within UCTD than in idiopathic interstitial pneumonia.

Histopathological finding. NSIP is characterized by interstitium expansion, which contains variable amounts on chronic inflammatory cellularization and fibrotization of various ages. Distribution of the changes is more diffuse without bronchiolocentric predominance or subpleural/paraseptal localization. Quite often we can find sections of organizing pneumonia, but these areas are not a dominant component of the affection. Fibrosis contains numerous collagen fibers as well as relatively numerous fibroblasts in contrast to UIP-IPF, where fibrotization contains only sporadic cells. In general, however, a fibrotic process makes an impression of the same age (so-called “time homogeneity”); fibroblastic focuses are present only sporadically or can be completely missing.

In case of IPF, the principal histomorphological feature in a small magnification is the focal affection of lung parenchyma. Areas affected by chronic interstitial inflammatory process and fibrosis containing fibroblastic focuses alternate with areas of relatively normal, unaffected lung parenchyma. Fibrotically changed lung parenchyma is infiltrated by relatively well-formed fibrosis that consists of only very little cellular, hyaline-transformed dense collagen connective tissue. Parts of granulation tissue with accumulation of fibroblasts with myxoid stroma directly link up with this old fibrotization. This considerable variability of the age of fibrotic changes (time heterogeneity) is typical for this type of affliction.

Case Report of Idiopathic Pulmonary Fibrosis That Was Not Idiopathic

A 69-year-old patient visited us on his own volition for the first time in 2011. Previously he had been under the care of a local pneumologist for 2 years due to idiopathic pulmonary fibrosis.

Family history: Mother died at age 71 from hematologic cancer; father died at age 78 after a head injury. He has two younger sisters who are healthy. Daughter is healthy as well, but son suffers from celiac disease. Both of son's children have celiac and are lactose intolerant. No pulmonary diseases have occurred in the family.

Past history: He had measles and pertussis in childhood, did not suffer from any other serious diseases as a child. At age 50, elevated cholesterol was detected during a routine examination and he began to take a hypolipidemic drug (Tulip). In 2007 severe arthrosis of the right hip joint was documented and he underwent implantation of a total endoprosthesis the same year. After the surgery he was diagnosed with arterial hypertension and he began to take Loradur Mite and Lozap. He has taken Pangrol for 10 years due to chronic pancreatitis. Ultrasonography was performed, without pathologic findings. He also underwent a colonoscopy with regard to celiac disease in the son and grandchildren; an asymptomatic polyp was removed during the examination. He has been hoarse for several years; only nodules on the vocal cords were found during the otorhinolaryngologic examination. Since the death of his wife (3 years ago) he has been taking Citalec for depression. He had unclear dysphagic problems in the past, which were probably esophageal spasm.

Social and working history, abuses: The patient is currently retired; he used to work as a service technician. He does not have any animals at home, lives in a flat in an apartment building. He used to smoke 20 cigarettes a day, but quit smoking 34 years ago.

Allergies: None.

Present complaint: After the hip replacement he began to notice dyspnea on exertion that has significantly worsened in the last 2 years. During the control orthopedic examination he was referred to a local pneumologist's office. He had a chest X-ray with subsequent chest HRCT scan that revealed pulmonary fibrosis. Bronchoalveolar lavage (BAL) and lung biopsy were not performed at that time, since the patient refused both tests. At that time, his wife died of pancreatic cancer and he was depressed. Therapy with *N*-acetylcysteine (Mucobene 2 × 600 mg) and Pentoxyphyllin (Pentomer R) was initiated at the recommendation of the hospital clinic. He continued to be cared for by the local pneumologist. In July 2011 he experienced significant worsening of the dyspnea, stopping many times while walking on a flat surface while carrying groceries. Medrol was prescribed – at first 16 mg daily and then later increased to 32 mg daily. Currently the dosage is 16 mg every other day. This therapy resulted in the appearance of diabetes mellitus that is currently being treated by oral antidiabetic agents, and the glaucoma is being treated topically by Timohexal. Spirometry was performed only at the time of diagnosis, when the vital capacity was 72 % of the predicted values; the diffusing capacity (DLco) and acid-base balance have never been examined. The condition has not improved after corticosteroid therapy. He still felt worse and therefore decided to visit our clinic. He agreed to additional tests, including BAL, and a possible lung transplantation if we proposed it.

Our Examination

Physical examination: The patient is slightly obese, hoarse, without icterus, cyanosis or drumstick fingers; auscultation: crepitus bilaterally to one half of scapulae, regular heart rhythm, two heart sounds without murmurs; abdomen without pathologic findings; lower extremities without edema or signs of inflammation.

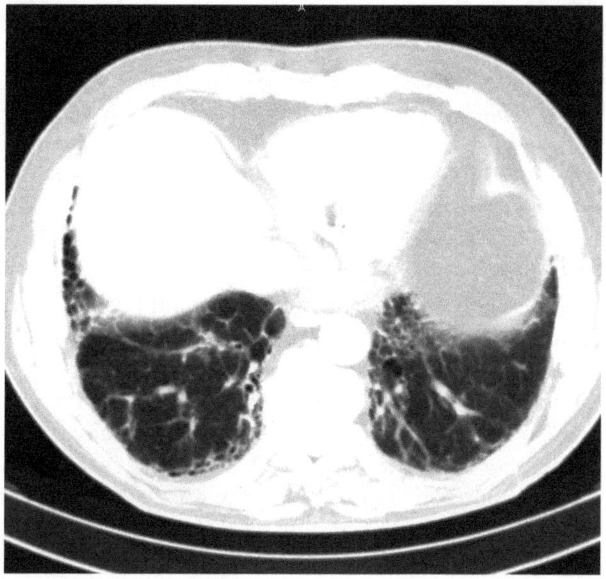

Fig. 1 HRCT finding compatible with the diagnosis of IPF-UIP with the fibrosis and areas of honeycomb lung in subpleural basal part, more pronounced on the *right* side

Chest X-ray: Skeleton without pathologic findings, heart silhouette of normal size and configuration, higher position of hemi-diaphragms bilaterally, reduced lung fields, coarse reticular changes bilaterally, most pronounced in basal parts.

Delivered description of *chest HRCT scan*: The finding is compatible with moderate idiopathic pulmonary fibrosis (IPF) (Fig. 1).

Spirometry: FVC 1.98 L (54 % of predicted value), FEV1 1.78 L (62 % of predicted value) – moderate restrictive ventilatory defect.

DLCO: 36 % of predicted value – markedly reduced.

Acid-base balance: pH: 7.486, pCO_2: 4.65, pO_2: 8.12 – mild hypoxemic respiratory insufficiency.

Spiroergometry: Exercise tolerance is decreased, predominantly due to mechanical limitation of ventilation; oxygenation decreases only insignificantly; high dead space at rest significantly decreases; circulation response is adequate with slow dynamics of SV; probability of pulmonary arterial hypertension is low. Mechanical defect is much more serious than the respiratory, which could mean a slightly better prognosis.

Bone densitometry: Without osteoporosis.

Fibrobronchoscopy: Local anesthesia with Tetracaine, Lidocaine. Fibroscope inserted in sitting position via mouth, cavum laryngis is free, vocal cords are symmetrical, motion intact. Trachea is free, main carina is sharp. Both bronchial trunks were inspected, orifices of segmental and subsegmental bronchi are free in visualized parts. Mucous membranes are pale.

Conclusion: Diffuse atrophic changes of mucous membranes; otherwise the findings are normal.

BAL was performed from the subsegment of the middle bronchus – 22, 23, 34, 32 mL, transbronchial biopsy from the bronchus of the lower right lobe was taken – five samples for histological examination.

The procedure was without any complications.

BAL fluid cytology: 69 % alveolar macrophages, 9 % neutrophil granulocytes, 16 % lymphocytes, 6 % eosinophil granulocytes.

Histopathological examination of transbronchial biopsy: The sample contains sections of bronchial wall covered by multi-layer ciliary epithelium of respiratory type with mild hyperplasia of goblet cells; under the slightly thickened basal membrane in subepithelial connective tissue is a mixed inflammatory infiltrate without marked participation of eosinophil granulocytes, with mild hyperplasia of smooth muscle. The sample contains relatively large pieces of peribronchial lung parenchyma as well. The dominant finding is marked peribronchial fibrotization with intense mixed inflammatory cellularity, which also spreads to widened interalveolar septa. We also documented interstitial and alveolar edema; additional sections also showed the apparent spreading of young collagen connective tissue and of organizing granulation tissue with the overall picture of organizing pneumonia. We also found scattered groups of siderophages. Conclusion: The sample generally does not provide unequivocal support for the diagnosis. Peribronchial lung parenchyma contains an apparent pattern of intense mixed inflammatory infiltration suggesting organizing pneumonia. Obvious signs of clinically assumed UIP have not been documented, but such or other biologically advanced processes can be located in an adjacent area.

Diagnosis and Treatment

On the basis of these tests, the patient was diagnosed with idiopathic pulmonary fibrosis, probably of usual type (UIP). Medical history, auscultation finding of crepitations and chest HRCT scan contributed the most to the diagnosis despite the fact that the bronchoscopic biopsy documented in particular the signs of organizing pneumonia and unspecified fibrosis, and BAL fluid contained not only neutrophil granulocytes and eosinophils, but also significantly higher numbers of lymphocytes. Therefore gradual withdrawal of the Medrol was recommended. Pentomer was also discontinued, Mucobene was increased to a recommended dosage of 3 × 600 mg and preventive anti-reflux therapy was added (Helicid 20 mg 2 × 1 tablet) as given in the most recent guidelines of the largest international pneumologic societies for IPF treatment. Anti-fibrotic therapy – Pirfenidone was also considered and an immunological exam was supplemented. With regard to IPF diagnosis and hypoxemic respiratory insufficiency, we also considered lung transplantation so we performed coronarography and heart catheterization. Only hemodynamically insignificant stenoses of coronary arteries not requiring intervention were found. Esophageal spasms have not been demonstrated during gastroenterological examination, including manometry. Since the end of 2011 the patient has been enrolled in a Pirfenidone therapeutic program, receiving a recommended daily dose of 3 × 3 capsules, i.e., 2,403 mg. daily. After only 3 months has this therapy led to a significant improvement in the subjective condition, and an improvement of the diffusing capacity from 39 to 49 % of the predicted value. A moderately reduced vital capacity persists. A chest HRCT scan documented stationary findings without signs of disease activity and progression during the previous 6 months. According to the results of immunological examination, secondary immunodeficiency is not present despite previous corticosteroid therapy. However, positivity of ANA 1/160 with homogeneous fluorescence is present, as well as positivity of anti-dsDNA antibodies and anti-topoisomerase antibodies.

Conclusion

We finalized the diagnosis as interstitial pneumonia of usual interstitial pneumonia type (UIP), probably within UCTD; idiopathic pulmonary fibrosis is less probable. With regard to the fact that clinical findings are not unambiguous for any systemic connective tissue disease, and the HRCT finding corresponds to UIP, we are continuing with anti-fibrotic treatment (Pirfenidone) together with Mucobene and Helicid. The patient's condition is stable with this treatment, currently without hypoxemic respiratory insufficiency and with improvement of functional parameters at the last visit (half a year after the initiation of treatment) to a moderately restrictive ventilatory defect. The diffusing capacity remains the same after a previous improvement.

Bibliography

1. Corte TJ, Copley SJ, Desai SR, Zapala CJ, Hansell DM, Nicholson AG, Colby TV, Renzoni E, Maher TM, Wells AU (2012) Significance of connective tissue disease features in idiopathic interstitial pneumonia. Eur Respir J 39:661–668
2. Tzelepis GE, Toya SP, Moutsopoulos HM (2008) Occult connective tissue diseases mimicking idiopathic interstitial pneumonias. Eur Respir J 31:11–20

Atypical Forms of Granulomatosis with Polyangiitis (Wegener's)

Jozef Rovenský

Contents

Discussion 46
References 48

Abstract

In this chapter we presented the occurrence of an atypical course of granulomatosis with polyangiitis (GPA) (formerly known as Wegener's granulomatosis), which can also be called a "limited form." Basically it is an incomplete manifestation of GPA that does not fulfill diagnostic criteria, but on the other hand the involvement of some of the organs can have a fatal outcome. An atypical course or limited form belongs to the group of sine syndromes in inflammatory rheumatic diseases that are not very common, but it is necessary to take them into account within differential diagnostics. An important aspect of the above-mentioned forms of GPA is its unusual course (involvement of uterine neck, compression of ureter, and other complications that can occur in these forms). We also give examples of the combination of Sjögren's syndrome with GPA as well as the incidence of this disease in young patients.

So-called atypical forms or sine syndromes can occur in inflammatory rheumatic diseases, in which a severe course can be present, while the disease does not fulfill diagnostic criteria. In our review we present current data from the literature on the occurrence of atypical forms of granulomatosis with polyangiitis (AF-GPA).

J. Rovenský
National Institute of Rheumatic Diseases, Piešťany, Slovakia

Institute of Physiotherapy, Balneology and Therapeutic Rehabilitation, University of Saint Cyril and Methodius, Trnava, Piešťany, Slovakia
e-mail: jozef.rovensky@nurch.sk

J. Rovensky et al. (eds.), *Sine Syndromes in Rheumatology*,
DOI 10.1007/978-3-7091-1541-1_7, © Springer-Verlag Wien 2014

Table 1 Overview of patients with atypical form of granulomatosis with polyangiitis

Publication year	Gender	Age	Diagnosis/ form	Localization	ANCA	Course
1985	Not given	Not given	Limited form of GPA	Skin, lips	Not given	
1994	Female	36	Protracted superficial GPA	Skin, lungs, mucosa	–	13-year duration of granulomatous ulcers before determining the diagnosis
2000	Female	44	Protracted superficial GPA	Skin, lungs, upper respiratory tract	Not given	10-year duration of subcutaneous nodes on lower extremities before the onset of systemic disease
2001	Female	47	Relapsing GPA	Skin, lungs, upper respiratory tract, kidneys	ANCA +	Complete remission for 20 years, death due to pneumonia 4 months after the disease relapse
2003	Female	74	Atypical cutaneous form	skin	ANCA –	Complete remission for 6 years, absence of systemic manifestations

Adopted from Kuchel and Lee [5–9]

Clinical findings in GPA consist of the triad of necrotizing granulomas in the upper and lower respiratory tracts, glomerulonephritis and generalized vasculitis.

Limited forms with pulmonary lesions, but without glomerulonephritis, can be considered AF-GPA [1]. Furthermore, it can be a protracted variant with necrotic ulcers localized primarily on the skin and in mucosa with a very mild course [2]. The disease can be present for several months or even years before the manifestation of the severe, multi-organ form of GPA. In a variant of GPA, the face is affected, while on the other hand, in the typical form of GPA, skin lesions occur also on the lower extremities [2, 3].

In the case of AF-GPA, it is more difficult to determine the diagnosis, since a nosographic demarcation of the disease is absent. However, the disease can be fatal if adequate therapy is not administered early enough [4].

Several patients with AF-GPA were documented in literature sources (Table 1).

Discussion

Granulomatosis with polyangiitis was described for the first time by F. Wegener in 1937 as a fatal multisystemic disease. It manifests as necrotizing granulomatosis that affects the respiratory tract; focal necrotizing vasculitis and focal necrotizing glomerulonephritis are also present. A typical feature of GPA is high mortality and morbidity. Carrington and Leibow [10] described a limited form of GPA without renal involvement, with a mild course and better prognosis. However, it is still not clear whether it is a separate nosologic entity or an early stage of the classic form of GPA [10]. Kakizawa et al. [11] presented the case of a 68-year-old woman who developed microscopic hematuria and proteinuria at age 50. She suffered from hearing impairment, arthralgia, retinal embolization, peripheral arterial occlusion of the right leg and chronic renal failure during the follow-up. At age 68, progressive renal failure with nephrotic syndrome and the presence of a high c-ANCA titer occurred. There were no signs of respiratory tract impairment. The administration of methylprednisolone pulse therapy and a low dosage of cyclophosphamide led to improvement of renal failure and reduction of the c-ANCA level, but the patient died on July 19,1998, due to fungal and *Pneumocystis carinii* infections. The absence of pulmonary symptoms suggests the atypical form of GPA; on the other hand, c-ANCA positivity that occurred in 1992, together with the clinical findings suggesting systemic vasculitis, confirm the diagnosis of GPA. From the point of view of other clinical symptoms in limited forms or AF-GPA, such as ophthalmic involvement, literature sources show that there can be the same incidence in limited as well as in classic forms. Retinal vascular occlusions can be the first manifestation of the disease, although it is uncommon. Only five cases with this manifestation of GPA were described between 1960 and 2002 [12].

From the other papers related to the problems of limited forms or AF-GPA, it is necessary to mention the paper of Krupsky et al. [13]. He presented a nodular form of GPA. Eosinophilia was found in peripheral blood as well as in pleural effusion. The patient responded very well to therapy with corticosteroids and cyclophosphamide. The above-mentioned variant of GPA is characterized by the absence of eosinophilia in lung parenchyma and a good response to immunosuppressive therapy.

Padhan et al. [14] presented an uncommon course of AF-GPA, where GPA occurred in a 15-year-old girl. The onset of the disease was manifested by acute renal failure on the basis of crescentic glomerulonephritis associated with the positivity of MPO-ANCA tests. Pulmonary hemorrhage and respiratory failure occurred 18 months later. A lung biopsy suggested GPA. The case showed the course of the disease initially manifested by crescentic glomerulonephritis with the presence of a perinuclear reaction (corresponding to p-ANCA presence). Later on, pulmonary hemorrhage with the development of pulmonary granulomas occurred. The authors state that the case is atypical because GPA does not occur in children and adolescents. The presence of atypical renal findings in the sense of ANCA-positive glomerulonephritis and relapse of pulmonary symptoms 18 months later is atypical. Before the initiation of constant immunosuppressive therapy, *Mycobacterium avium intracellulare* was found in a bronchoalveolar lavage. After recurrent hemorrhagic events, the patient received anti-TB treatment for 2 months and corticosteroids were discontinued.

Chang and Kerr [15] followed a patient with bilateral resistant uveitis and abdominal angina, with c-ANCA positivity. Despite a follow-up for 8 years, an angiographic exam was the one to confirm the presence of vasculitis and the patient subsequently received immunosuppressive therapy. The authors were convinced that it was an atypical course of GPA-type polyarteritis.

A limited form of AF-GPA can occur in connection with Sjögren's syndrome [16]. In a 60-year-old woman, dyspnea occurred for 5–6 weeks. A chest X-ray and CT scan suggested bilateral reticulonodular markings with the presence of c-ANCA, ANA and anti-Ro antibodies. A positive Schirmer's test and scintigraphy of salivary glands were clinical signs suggesting Sjögren's syndrome. A lung biopsy suggested granulomatous inflammation with multiple nuclear giant cells that infiltrated the lung parenchyma and vascular structures. Pathologic changes in the upper respiratory tract and kidneys were not observed. The diagnosis suggested a limited-pulmonary form of GPA and the presence of primary Sjögren's syndrome.

The limited form or AF-GPA can also be complicated by secondary infection. Shah et al. [17] described an AF-GPA relapse that was associated with occult nasal inflammation in the carrier (*Staphylococcus aureus*) of a 79-year-old female patient in whom a recurrent sclerotizing orbital pseudotumor complicated by an abscess occurred. The abscess was caused by *Streptococcus anginosis* (Milleri group). It was assumed that the secondary infection was responsible for the GPA exacerbation. Lillaz et al. [18] presented the fact that GPA can be one of the many causes of ureteral stenosis, i.e., the cause of the stenosis can be extra-urologic, while the other organs are not affected. The involvement of the uterine neck associated with intermenstrual bleeding is rare [19]. Clinical findings also included recurrent scleritis, arthralgia, weakness, nose crusts, obstruction and halitosis, saddle nose and perforation of nasal septum. A nasal biopsy showed active inflamed granulations with the presence of giant cells that are compatible with GPA despite the absence of granulomas and vasculitis. Laboratory parameters showed mildly elevated ESR and CRP values, and c-ANCA antibodies were moderately elevated.

References

1. Cassan SM, Coles DT, Harrison EG Jr (1970) The concept of limited forms of Wegener's granulomatosis. Am J Med 49:366–379
2. Hisler BM, Saltzman L (1991) Cutaneous involvement in Wegener's granulomatosis. Cutis 48:460–461
3. Hu C, O'Toughlin S, Winkelmann RK (1977) Cutaneous manifestations of Wegener's granulomatosis. Arch Dermatol 113:175–182
4. Chyu JY, Hagstrom WJ, Soltani K et al (1984) Wegener's granulomatosis in childhood: cutaneous manifestations as the presenting signs. J Am Acad Dermatol 10:341–346
5. Kihiczak D, Nychay SG, Schwartz RA et al (1994) Protracted superficial Wegener's granulomatosis. J Am Acad Dermatol 30:863–866
6. Kuchel J, Lee S (2003) Cutaneous Wegener's granulomatosis: a variant or atypical localized form? Australas J Dermatol 44:129–135
7. Hansen LS, Silverman S Jr, Pons VG et al (1985) Limited Wegener's granulomatosis. Report of a case with oral, renal, and skin involvement. Oral Surg Oral Med Oral Pathol 60:524–531
8. Figarella I, Bazarbachi T, Marie B et al (2000) Cutaneous nodules recurring in the legs ten years before the diagnosis of Wegener's granulomatosis. Rev Med Interne 21:693–697
9. Foltz V, Koeger AC, de Sauverzac C et al (2001) Relapse of Wegener's granulomatosis. Concerning a case after 20 years of remission. Joint Bone Spine 68:262–266

10. Carrington CB, Leibow AA (1966) Limited form of angiitis and granulomatosis of the Wegener's type. Am J Med 41:497–527
11. Kakizawa T, Ichikawa K, Yamauchi K et al (1999) Atypical Wegener's granulomatosis with positive cytoplasmic antineutrophil cytoplasmic antibodies, ophthalmologic manifestations, and slowly progressive renal failure without respiratory tract involvement. Intern Med 38(8):679–681
12. Shenoy R, Elagib el NM, al Siyabi H et al (2002) Limited Wegener's granulomatosis presenting as multiple retinal vascular occlusions. Indian J Ophthalmol 50(2):135–137
13. Krupsky M, Landau Z, Lifschitz-Mercer B et al (1993) Wegener's granulomatosis with peripheral eosinophilia. Chest 104:1290–1292
14. Pradhan M, Meyers KEC, Guttenberg M et al (2000) Wegener granulomatosis – an atypical case. Pediatr Nephrol 14:862–871
15. Chang YJ, Kerr LD (2000) Isolated abdominal vasculitis as an atypical presentation of Wegener's granulomatosis. Am J Gastroenterol 95(1):297–298
16. Yazisiz V, Ozbudak IH, Nizam I et al (2010) A case of primary Sjogren's syndrome with pulmonary-limited Wegener's granulomatosis. Rheumatol Int 30:1235–1238
17. Shah SA, Meyer DR, Foulke L et al (2010) Limited Wegener granulomatosis of the orbit complicated by Streptococcus anginosis (milleri group) infection. Grand Rounds 10:95–102
18. Lillaz J, Bernardini S, Algros MP et al (2011) Wegener's granulomatosis: a rare cause of hydronephrosis. Case Rep Med 2011:814794. doi:10.1155/2011/814794
19. Mukherjee S, Al-Utayem W, Bergin L et al (2011) Wegener's granulomatosis presenting as intermenstrual bleeding. J Obstet Gynaecol 31:191–192

Granulomatosis with Polyangiitis – Formerly Known as Wegener's Granulomatosis with Limited Manifestation Affecting Only Respiratory System

Martina Vašáková

Contents

Introduction 52
Examinations Aimed at Respiratory Tract in Suspected GPA 52
Treatment of Isolated Involvement of Respiratory Tract in GPA 55
Case Report of a Patient with Limited Pulmonary Involvement in GPA 56
Treatment and Follow-up 57
Conclusion 58
Bibliography 58

Abstract

Granulomatosis with polyangiitis (GPA), formerly known as Wegener's granulomatosis, is the most frequently occurring ANCA-associated vasculitis. As clinically incomplete, limited forms, we encounter relatively frequently with respiratory tract involvement, and not so rarely without the involvement of the lower respiratory tract or with minimal nose or ear symptoms. Positivity of antineutrophil cytoplasmic antibodies (ANCA) can be missing in isolated lung involvement. Patients with limited pulmonary involvement have a better prognosis than those with manifested renal involvement. DAH is a serious condition and only rarely does it occur without simultaneous renal involvement. Patients with limited involvement of the upper and lower respiratory tracts and lungs without DAH have a significantly better prognosis.

M. Vašáková
Department of Respiratory Medicine,
Thomayer University Hospital with Polyclinic, First Faculty of Medicine,
Charles University, Prague, Czech Republic
e-mail: martina.vasakova@ftn.cz

J. Rovensky et al. (eds.), *Sine Syndromes in Rheumatology*,
DOI 10.1007/978-3-7091-1541-1_8, © Springer-Verlag Wien 2014

Introduction

Granulomatosis with polyangiitis (GPA), formerly known as Wegener's granulomatosis, is the most frequently occurring ANCA-associated vasculitis.

Clinical presentation. In typical cases, GPA is commonly characterized by the following triad of symptoms:

1. Upper respiratory tract (epistaxis, sinusitis, otitis, ulcerations of mucous membranes, otalgia, mastoiditis, hearing loss, bone deformations, perforation of nasal septum, subglottic or bronchial stenoses)
2. Lower respiratory tract (cough, chest pain, dyspnea, hemoptysis)
3. Glomerulonephritis

However, not all of the signs have to be manifested at the time of diagnosis; renal involvement is present in less than 40 % of patients at the time of diagnosis, but it occurs in 90 % of patients in the course of the untreated disease. Systemic signs, ophtalmologic signs (keratoconjunctivitis, scleritis, uveitis, vasculitis and compression of optic nerve), as well as neurologic, dermatologic and musculoskeletal signs can also occur. General signs such as fatigue, weakness, fever and weight loss occur in 30–50 % of patients with GPA.

As clinically incomplete, limited forms, we encounter relatively frequently either with solitary respiratory tract involvement, without signs of kidney disease and sometimes even without involvement of upper respiratory tract. Positivity of anti-neutrophil cytoplasmic antibodies (ANCA) can be missing as well in these limited pulmonary manifestations of GPA.

From the clinical point of view we distinguish several possible types of respiratory tract involvement in GPA:

- Diffuse alveolar hemorrhage (DAH) (Fig. 1)
- Deforming or ulcerous lesions in upper and lower respiratory tracts (Fig. 2)
- Cavitary or nodular lesions that can be misinterpreted as abscessing pneumonia or tumor on X-rays (Fig. 3)

Examinations Aimed at Respiratory Tract in Suspected GPA

Pulmonary function tests. Spirometry. A ventilatory defect can be, but does not have to be present; central obstruction can be dominant in the case of lesions on large respiratory airways. If parenchyma is involved, we observe lower diffusion; on the contrary, diffusion increases in diffuse alveolar hemorrhage.

Laboratory examinations. Sideropenic anemia is usually present. In the case of renal involvement, we notice hematuria, proteinuria and signs of renal insufficiency. We can detect serum c-ANCA antibodies in the majority of patients with untreated GPA.

Otorhinolaryngologic examination. Despite the fact that the changes in the upper respiratory tract can be typical, histological findings are mostly non-specific, showing necrosis and inflammation.

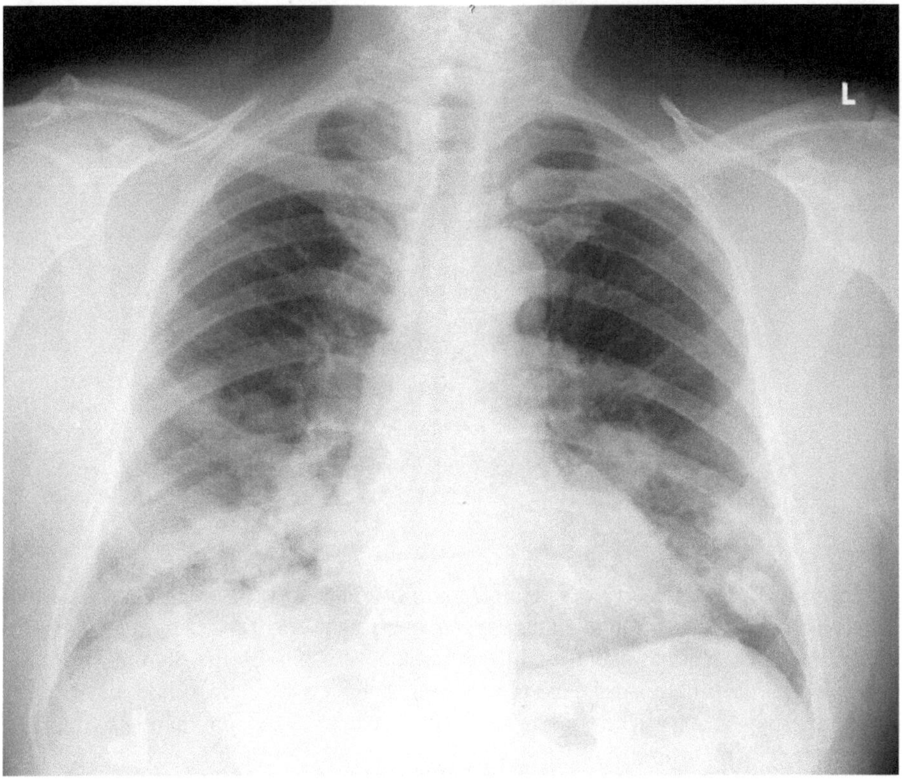

Fig. 1 Chest X-ray in a patient suffering from GPA with multiple pulmonary involvement with pulmonary cavitations

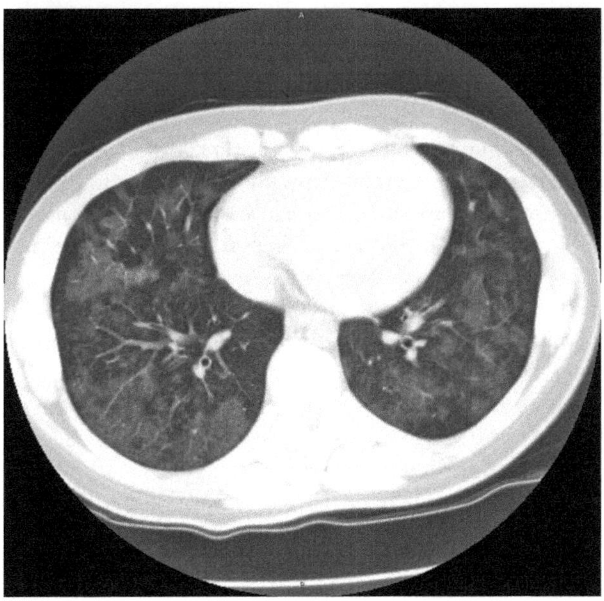

Fig. 2 Chest HRCT scan in a patient with GPA presenting as DAH

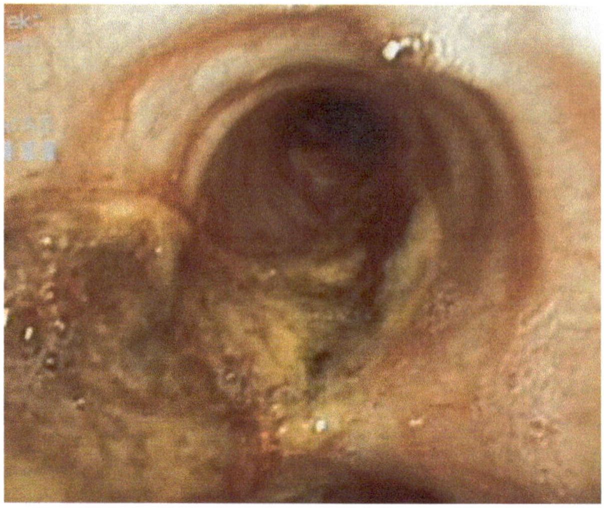

Fig. 3 Bronchoscopic finding in a patient with GPA with ulcerous lesion in the left main bronchus and at the carina of trachea

Imaging Methods. Skiagraphy or CT scan of upper respiratory tract and paranasal sinuses reveals pathologic changes in as many as 80 % of the patients with GPA.

Chest X-ray. Round, usually well-demarcated nodes with the diameter ranging from several millimeters to 10 cm are present. They are multiple, bilateral, and only rarely are they solitary. They can be located anywhere in the lung parenchyma. The nodes decay in one-third to one-half of the patients; arisen cavities have thick walls, are irregular with vanishing internal contour, and sometimes a hydroaeric phenomenon is present. They can change to cystic areas with thin walls over time. As a consequence of secondary pneumonic infiltrates or bleeding from vascular erosions, poorly demarcated or homogenous condensations can arise. Endobronchial changes can result in atelectasis of a lobe or of the whole lung (Fig. 1).

HRCT. Multiple nodes or masses with sharp irregular contours, often with a decay cavity are present; peripheral condensations of parenchyma can mimic pulmonary infarction. Calcifications are absent. Lesions are located along peripheral bronchovascular structures, without craniocaudal predilection. Ground glass opacities are also present. "Feeding vessel sign" is a frequent finding. "Halo sign" with ground glass opacity around hyperdense nodes can also occur (Fig. 2).

Bronchoscopy can reveal stenoses of large airways or ulcerous lesions (Fig. 3). We can also take the material for histological diagnosis (excision from the lesions or transbronchial biopsy). Transbronchial biopsy is usually not beneficial because the samples that it yields are too small. Bronchoalveolar lavage supports the diagnosis if the picture of DAH is present; there is progressive blood coloration during the return of individual portions of BAL fluid and we can subsequently identify hemosiderin-filled macrophages in cytological examinations of the fluid.

Histopathological examination. Pulmonary lesions in granulomatosis with polyangiitis in common magnification correspond to X-ray findings. The classical finding is a nodous consolidation of lung parenchyma with necrotization zones of various sizes, even of a geographic character. The principal diagnostic criteria include parenchyma necrosis, vasculitis and granulomatous inflammatory reaction. Granulomatous formations are typically associated with multinucleated giant cells, mostly of the foreign body type, that occur individually or in small groups. Less frequently, we can observe individual epitheloid granulomas of the sarcoid type; when found, it is always necessary to rule out necrotizing sarcoid granulomatosis. The finding of granulomatous formations not coupled with necrotic tissue also has to warrant a targeted search for infectious agents. Vasculitis in GPA typically affects small arteries and veins up to 5 mm in diameter. Except for the above-mentioned typical diagnostic changes, there is a big variety of accompanying histomorphological changes, such as alveolar hemorrhage, interstitial fibrosis, lipoid pneumonia, organizing pneumonia, hyperplasia of lymphoid elements, infiltration by eosinophil granulocytes, and xanthogranulomatous lesions. Respiratory airways can also be affected in the form of chronic bronchiolitis, acute bronchiolitis spreading to adjacent parenchyma, and even escalating to acute catarrhal-purulent bronchopneumonia, a picture of obliterative bronchiolitis with surrounding organizing pneumonia, bronchocentric granulomatosis, follicular bronchiolitis, or bronchial stenosis. In some cases the above-mentioned histopathological findings can dominate the diagnostic changes and they considerably complicate the determination of the correct diagnosis. For example, a picture of organizing pneumonia can be found in more than 70 % of biopsies obtained from patients with GPA. There are even cases when we do not find any other changes in a lung biopsy and a clinical + radiological picture of the disease is relatively typical. The specific term "organizing pneumonia-like variant of granulomatosis with polyangiitis" is used for such a finding.

Histopathological signs of organ involvement in GPA are often very convincing; however, it is always inevitable to correlate the micro-morphological picture with clinical and radiological findings and serological data before determining the definitive diagnosis.

Treatment of Isolated Involvement of Respiratory Tract in GPA

1. We use the classic combination of prednisone at a 1 mg/kg initial dose combined with cyclophosphamide at a 1 mg/kg daily dose for the treatment of GPA without DAH. Corticosteroids are successively withdrawn within 9 months and the overall duration of the treatment should be 12–18 months. After 3–6 months we can replace cyclophosphamide with azathioprine, mycophenolate mofetil or methotrexate. Trimethoprim/sulfamethoxazole 160/800 mg twice daily can be used in limited pulmonary involvement of a small extent and in anti-relapse therapy.
2. Urgent methylprednisolone pulse therapy (1 g intravenously for 3 days) is indicated in DAH. Sometimes we also indicate plasmapheresis in an acute phase.
3. Biological therapy targeted against CD4+ T-lymphocytes, B-lymphocytes (anti-CD20) and against cytokins (TNF-alpha) is also studied. From these novel therapies it is worth mentioning rituximab – an anti-CD20 antibody that probably

causes not only the depletion of B-lymphocytes and thus the formation of autoantibodies, but also affects the regulation roles of T- and B-lymphocytes.

Prognosis. Patients with limited pulmonary involvement have a better prognosis than those with manifested renal involvement. DAH is a serious condition and only rarely does it occur without simultaneous renal involvement. Patients with limited involvement of the upper and lower respiratory tracts and lungs without DAH have a significantly better prognosis.

Case Report of a Patient with Limited Pulmonary Involvement in GPA

A 25-year-old male patient was referred by an otorhinolaryngologist at the end of 2011.

Family history: Mother suffers from thyropathy; father is healthy, as are siblings. He does not have any children. Cousin suffers from type 1 diabetes.

Social and working history, abuses: He studies economics at the university. He has never smoked or taken drugs.

Past history: He had surgery for testicular torsion at age 9. He has not experienced any other serious illnesses.

Present complaint: He was examined in Olomouc due to chronic rhinitis in 2010. He underwent a biopsy of nasal mucous membrane at the Department of Otorhinolaryngology that was diagnosed as GPA. Chest X-ray was initially performed, and no pathologic changes were found. Bronchoscopy was not carried out. Positivity of anti-neutrophil cytoplasmic antibodies (c-ANCA) was confirmed from the onset of the disease. Later on he was treated by a rheumatologist with systemic corticosteroids in the form of monotherapy and due to local nasal findings without any improvement he was repeatedly referred to the Department of Otorhinolaryngology. Despite corticosteroid therapy, the patient experienced secretion from the right, and later on from the left ear, at the beginning of 2011. *Staphylococcus aureus* was confirmed in the cultures. He underwent local treatment and had autovaccines administered at the Department of Otorhinolaryngology. He was referred by otorhinolaryngologist to our clinic due to a cough and hemoptysis in December 2012. At that time he was on Medrol therapy, alternating 2- and 4-mg daily doses.

Our Examination. Physical examination: saddle nose, rhinolalia, lungs: vesicular clean breathing, regular heart rhythm, two heart sounds without murmurs, abdomen without pathologic findings, lower extremities without edema or signs of inflammation.

Laboratory results: renal parameters in reference range, ANCA IF positivity (ELISA-MPOA: 1.4, PR3A: > 150)

Radiological findings:

Chest X-ray: focal change with translucency in upper left lung lobe of 6 cm in diameter.

Chest CT scan: decay cavity in the left upper lobe with thick walls and hydroaeric phenomenon located in subpleural area, left-sided hilar lymphadenopathy.

Bronchoscopy: Apparent ulceration on the ventral wall of larynx and in subglottic area with inflammatory changes in adjacent mucous membranes, infiltrated mucous membrane with fine granulations and erosions in the left main bronchus; otherwise normal endobronchial finding. Bronchoscopic changes are compatible with the involvement of larynx and large airways in GPA.

Transbronchial biopsy from the focus in the left lung: Histopathological findings: Observed changes correlated to positivity of ANCA antibodies corresponding to granulomatosis with a high probability of polyangiitis.

Otorhinolaryngologic examination: Otoscopic examination: tympanic membrane with the injection in manubrium area, otherwise normal findings on the right side. Left tympanic membrane is retracted, matte, light reflex present, without secretion. Rhinoscopic examination: nasal mucous membrane is bleeding bilaterally, crusts are present bilaterally, septum is perforated.

Nephrologic examination: Only isolated erythrocyturia without signs of renal involvement according to ultrasonography; renal biopsy was not indicated.

On the basis of the extent of the disease (major affection of upper and lower respiratory tract, large decay cavity in the left lung, extreme values of anti-PR3 ANCA) we offered and recommended to the patient combined immunosuppressive therapy – cyclophosphamide (600 mg) pulse therapy in 4-week intervals together with an initial increase of the corticosteroid dosage. The patient did not agree to this procedure and returned to the rheumatologist who increased the dosage of systemic corticosteroids to 32 mg daily and sent the application for rituximab approval to the health insurance company. Despite the increased corticosteroid dosage, the patient returned in a month with recurrent hemoptysis and intermittent subfebrilities.

Radiological changes in the left lung: Chest X-ray showed progression of cavity size to 10×6 cm.

Lung function tests: Spirometry values: FVC: 6.11 L (106 % of predicted value), FEV1: 5.19 L (107 % of predicted value), diffusion: 97 % of predicted value – within reference range.

Treatment and Follow-up

The patient was informed that the refusal of combined immunosuppressive therapy or its postponement could result in life-threatening complications (risk of severe lung hemorrhage, destruction of larynx structures). The patient did not agree to hospitalization; however, he consented to out-patient administration of immunosuppressive therapy. Before its initiation the patient was referred to the Center for Assisted Reproduction for sperm storage. On February 8th, 2012, we started with cyclophosphamide pulse therapy as mentioned above, and initially continued with a 32 mg dose of Medrol. We decreased the dosage of Medrol to 16 mg daily from March. The patient's subjective condition considerably improved, chest X-ray confirmed basically complete regression of decay cavity in the left lung (after the second pulse of cyclophosphamide). Co-trimoxazole 960 mg daily divided into two doses was added to the therapy, as well as Calcichew D3 once daily for osteoporosis prevention.

Check-up bronchoscopy after third pulse of Cyclophosphamide: regression of ulcerative lesions in larynx, trachea and the left main bronchus.

The dosage of systemic corticosteroids continued to be decreased; six pulses of cyclophosphamide were administered as scheduled, with the last on July 4th, 2012. Subsequently the patient was switched to azathioprine 150 mg daily, divided into three doses together with medrol 8 mg daily and co-trimoxazole as long-term preventive therapy. The patient feels well, X-ray and bronchoscopy confirmed complete regression of the changes in the larynx, trachea and lung parenchyma. An otorhinolaryngologic exam showed a milder form of persistent nasal mucous membrane involvement and perforation of nasal septum. ANCA-IF positivity persists, but PR3A titers have decreased significantly, from >150 to 14.4. Other autoantibodies are negative.

Conclusion

In this patient, GPA affecting only the respiratory tract was concluded, but with a major, multilocular progressive involvement of airways as well as of lung parenchyma. The diagnosis was formulated as follows:

ANCA-positive vasculitis of GPA type (formerly known as Wegener's granulomatosis) with ENT involvement (atrophic crustous rhinopharyngitis, nasal septum perforation, otitis media secretorica, *Staphylococcus aureus* colonization), ulcerations on the ventral wall of the larynx and in the subglottic area with inflammatory changes in adjacent mucous membranes and pulmonary involvement (granuloma in the left lung with central decay), without renal involvement.

It can be concluded that in vasculitis, and especially in GPA-WG, it is always necessary to search for the extent of organ involvement. Respiratory tract involvement, either in the form of the upper and large lower respiratory tract or lung parenchyma involvement is very frequent and commonly occurs without any other disease manifestations. Bronchoscopy and chest X-ray (also repeated ones) are inevitable at the onset of the disease and before initiation of treatment, but also during further check-ups. We adjust the therapy to the severity of respiratory tract involvement. In the case of diffuse alveolar hemorrhage or multilocular involvement with high ANCA titers, combined immunosuppressive therapy is indicated, while in limited forms it is possible to try the therapy with co-trimoxazole alone.

Bibliography

Frankel SK, Cosgrove GP, Fischer A, Meehan RT, Brown KK (2006) Update in the diagnosis and management of pulmonary vasculitis. Chest 129:452–465

Vasculitis with Thrombosis

Manfred Herold

Contents

Case Report No. 1 60
Case Report No. 2 61
Case Report No. 3 61
Case Report No. 4 62
References 62

Abstract

Vasculitis is an inflammation of the blood vessel wall causing damage to the wall followed by a wide variety of signs and symptoms, depending on the type of vessels and organs affected. Inflammation-caused vessel wall injury leads to vascular stenosis, occlusion, aneurysm and bleeding. Thrombosis is not a common symptom but may occur, resulting in serious complications in various conditions of vasculitis.

Abbreviations

AAV	ANCA-associated vasculitis
ANCA	Anti-neutrophil cytoplasmic antibodies
CRP	C-reactive protein
CSS	Churg-Strauss Syndrome
EPA	Eosinophilic granulomatosis with polyangiitis

M. Herold, MD, PhD
Rheumatology Unit, Department of Internal Medicine VI,
Innsbruck Medical University, Anichstrasse 35,
Innsbruck, Tirol A-6020, Austria
e-mail: manfred.herold@i-med.ac.at

J. Rovensky et al. (eds.), *Sine Syndromes in Rheumatology*,
DOI 10.1007/978-3-7091-1541-1_9, © Springer-Verlag Wien 2014

ESR	Erythrocyte sedimentation rate
GPA	Granulomatosis with polyangiitis
PE	Pulmonary embolism
VTE	Venous thromboembolism

Vasculitis is characterized by injury to a vessel wall caused by inflammation. Vasculitis can affect arteries, veins, and capillaries. The clinical manifestations depend on the type and size of the affected blood vessels. Damage to the vessel wall may result in stenosis with diminished blood flow, obstruction followed by necrosis, aneurism with danger of rupture and sudden bleeding, or it may result in widespread bleeding as a result of the leakage of the vessel wall.

Vasculitis is a rare disease that affects people of both sexes and all ages. Some types of vasculitis occur in certain age groups more often than in others. The clinical signs depend on the size, number and location of the involved blood vessels.

There are more than 20 different disorders that are classified as "vasculitis." The nomenclature follows the recommendations of the International Chapel Hill Consensus Conference, which published revised criteria in 2013 [1]. The group of vasculitides includes many different types of diseases that are similar in some ways, but often differ with respect to affected organs, medications used in treatment, and other characteristics. Though vasculitis is a term for a group of rare diseases, there are many different types of vasculitis, which may vary greatly in symptoms, severity and duration. Finding the correct diagnosis [2] and starting the recommended treatment as soon as possible is the primary goal in the management of patients with vasculitis.

Thromboembolic disease is not expected as a main feature in vasculitis but is an increasingly recognized complication of several vasculitides [3, 4]. Inflammation and coagulation are closely related to each other [5]. It is commonly observed that thromboembolic complications coincide with periods of increased vasculitis disease activity. The underlying mechanisms causing this are still not known. In large- and medium-vessel vasculitis, thrombosis may result in stenosis and occlusion. In ANCA-associated vasculitis (AAV) and in Behcet's disease, the risk for venous thrombotic events seems to be increased. In AAV, thrombosis is associated with increased disease activity [4].

In a retrospective review of 19 patients with eosinophilic granulomatosis with polyangiitis (EPA; Churg-Strauss Syndrome), thrombosis was a significant complication and authors conclude that thromboprophylaxis may be warranted in EPA [6]. When managing patients with vasculitis, questions remain about the screening of asymptomatic patients, prevention of thrombosis, and duration of anticoagulation if treatment has already begun [7].

Case Report No. 1 [8]

A 61-year-old woman was diagnosed with AAV-type GPA (Wegener's granulomatosis) 24 months ago with nasal inflammation, abnormal chest radiography and granulomatosis inflammation on a lung biopsy; she had been in remission for

18 months under treatment with prednisolone (10 mg/day) and sulfamethoxazole. She came to the emergency unit with a seven-day history of left-leg edema, purpura on both legs and dyspnea and hemoptysis for three days. An ancillary test revealed elevated erythrocyte sedimentation rate, cANCA positivity and pulmonary embolism with pulmonary infarction and deep vein thrombosis. Consequently, the patient received a diagnosis of ANCA-associated vasculitis with venous thromboembolism (VTE). Therapy was started with enoxaparin, higher doses of prednisolone, cyclophosphophamide, sulfamethoxazole and oxygen. However, two days later the patient suddenly died. The circumstances of her death were consistent with the occurrence of another PE.

Conclusion: Pulmonologists should consider the possibility of VTE in active ANCA-associated vasculitis.

Case Report No. 2 [9]

A 64-year-old woman was admitted to the hospital with angina and signs of heart failure of 2 weeks' duration. The patient had a flu-like illness 3 months before, followed by fatigue, malaise, arthralgia, myalgia, orthostatic dizziness, and morning stiffness. Symptoms improved in response to oral diclofenac. On admission, an ECG showed ST-T changes but no pathological changes were seen in echocardiography. Blood tests revealed ESR 90 mm/h and CRP 16.5 mg/L. Over the next few days, patient presented with fever and increasing shortness of breath. Among other tests and imaging procedures, an open lung biopsy was taken and revealed histological signs of neutrophilic microabscesses, thrombosis, hemorrhage and granuloma characteristic for GPA (Wegener's granulomatosis). After diagnosis of GPA, intravenous methylprednisolone and oral cyclophosphamide were initiated. The patient was able to be discharged 3 weeks later with oral medication.

Conclusion: The initial diagnostic confusion was due to the oligosymptomatic presentation (limited GPA) with angina and signs of heart failure and underlines the fact that GPA can present with myocardial ischemia due to coronary vasculitis, primarily in small- and medium-sized coronary arteries at the cardiac apex.

Case Report No. 3 [10]

A 58-year-old man was admitted to the otorhinolaryngology department because of a sudden swelling and erythema of the left parotid gland that did not respond to antibiotic treatment. Blood tests were unremarkable except for elevated ESR (89 mm/h) and CRP (50 mg/L). A biopsy of the parotid gland revealed a necrotizing parotitis. A chest X-ray and computed tomography were consistent with bilateral pleural effusion and bilateral pulmonary infiltrates and nodules. Immunology tests showed the presence of cANCA with anti-PR3 specifity. Three weeks later the patient developed hemoptysis and right leg edema due to a right femoral vein thrombosis. The work-up for the hypercoagulability state resulted in a strong positivity for a lupus coagulant. Therapeutic procedures included plasmapheresis, hemodialysis, intravenous cyclophosphamide and methylprednisolone. The patient was able to be discharged with oral medication and presented in clinical remission at a visit 4 months later.

Conclusion: Vasculitis does not exclude the incidence with other serious syndromes. This case shows an unusual presentation of generalized GPA starting as necrotizing isolated parotitis and accompanied by a life-threatening APS.

Case Report No. 4 [11]

A 35-year-old Turkish man presented with facial swelling and visible dilated collateral veins over the thorax. These symptoms had begun 3 months prior to his admission. Besides a history of symptoms typical of Behcet's disease, he also reported deep vein thrombosis in his calf. ESR was 51 mm/h, CRP 145 mg/L. Echocardiography and computed tomography showed extensive thrombosis of the superior vena cava with multiple collateral vascular structures in the mediastinum secondary to the occlusion of the superior vena cava. He was diagnosed with Behcet's disease based on typical clinical features including thrombophlebitis in the absence of any other specific etiology. Immunosuppressive therapies, together with oral anticoagulants, were the treatment of choice.

Conclusion: Behcet' syndrome is a multisystem vascultits of unknown etiology and a unique geographic distribution. It may involve all sizes and types of vessels. Lower extremity vein thrombosis is the most frequent manifestation of vascular involvement followed by vena cava thrombosis and other symptoms [12, 13].

References

1. Jennette JC, Falk RJ, Bacon PA, Basu N, Cid MC, Ferrario F, Flores-Suarez LF, Gross WL, Guillevin L, Hagen EC, Hoffman GS, Jayne DR, Kallenberg CG, Lamprecht P, Langford CA, Luqmani RA, Mahr AD, Matteson EL, Merkel PA, Ozen S, Pusey CD, Rasmussen N, Rees AJ, Scott DG, Specks U, Stone JH, Takahashi K, Watts RA (2013) 2012 Revised International Chapel Hill Consensus Conference Nomenclature of Vasculitides. Arthritis Rheum 65:1–11
2. Konttinen YT, Rotar Z, Pettersson T, Nordström DC, Bacon P, Petersen J (2006) Roadmap to vasculitis. Acta Reumatol Port 31:15–36
3. Gaffo AL (2013) Thrombosis in vasculitis. Best Pract Res Clin Rheumatol 27:57–67
4. Tomasson G, Monach PA, Merkel PA (2009) Thromboembolic disease in vasculitis. Curr Opin Rheumatol 21:41–46
5. Tichelaar YI, Kluin-Nelemans HJ, Meijer K (2012) Infections and inflammatory diseases as risk factors for venous thrombosis. A systematic review. Thromb Haemost 107:827–837
6. Whyte AF, Smith WB, Sinkar SN, Kette FE, Hissaria P (2013) Clinical and laboratory characteristics of nineteen patients with Churg-Strauss syndrome from a single South Australian centre. Intern Med J. 43:784–790. doi:10.1111/imj.12173
7. Springer J, Villa-Forte A (2013) Thrombosis in vasculitis. Curr Opin Rheumatol 25:19–25
8. Santana AN, Takagaki TY, Barbas CS (2011) Incidence of fatal venous thromboembolism in antineutrophil cytoplasmic antibody-associated vasculitis. J Bras Pneumol 37:409–411
9. Cocco G, Gasparyan AY (2010) Myocardial ischemia in Wegener's granulomatosis: coronary atherosclerosis versus vasculitis. Open Cardiovasc Med J 4:57–62

10. Shovman O, Langevitz P, Gilburd B, Shoenfeld Y (2013) Coincidence of granulomatosis and polyangiitis with atypical clinical manifestation and antiphospholipid syndrome. Lupus 22:320–323
11. Solmaz D, Sari I, Ozpelit E, Yilmaz E (2011) Intracardiac thrombosis and superior vena cava syndrome in Behçet's disease. Intern Med 50:1787–1788
12. Seyahi E, Yurdakul S (2011) Behçet's syndrome and thrombosis. Mediterr J Hematol Infect Dis 3(1):e2011026. doi:10.4084/MJHID.2011.026
13. La Regina M, Gasparyan AY, Orlandini F, Prisco D (2010) Behçet's disease as a model of venous thrombosis. Open Cardiovasc Med J 4:71–77

Atypical Course of Rheumatoid Arthritis

Jozef Rovenský, Dagmar Mičeková, Zlata Kmečová, Mária Stančíková, Jindřiška Gatterová, Martina Vašáková, Jana Sedláková, Peter Poprac, and Alena Tuchyňová

Contents

Case Report No. 1: Absence of Erosive Changes on X-Rays in Spite of 20-Year Duration of Rheumatoid Arthritis 66
Case Report No. 2: Rheumatoid Arthritis with Dominating Pulmonary Involvement and Oligosymptomatic Articular Involvement 67
Discussion 71
References 73

Abstract

Rheumatoid arthritis is an inflammatory disease characterized by the involvement of peripheral joints with the development of erosive changes on X-rays of the affected joints. In some cases, the disease can run an atypical course. In the following case reports, we present a patient with rheumatoid arthritis who, despite the disease lasting for several years with high clinical activity, did not

J. Rovenský (✉) • D. Mičeková • P. Poprac
National Institute of Rheumatic Diseases, Piešťany, Slovakia

Institute of Physiotherapy, Balneology and Therapeutic Rehabilitation, University of Saint Cyril and Methodius, Trnava, Piešťany, Slovakia
e-mail: jozef.rovensky@nurch.sk

Z. Kmečová
Rheumatology Outpatients Department, Roosevelt Hospital, Banská Bystrica, Slovakia

M. Stančíková • J. Sedláková • A. Tuchyňová
National Institute of Rheumatic Diseases, Nábrežie I. Krasku 4, Piešťany 921 12, Slovakia

J. Gatterová
Institute of Rheumatology, Prague, Czech Republic

M. Vašáková
Department of Respiratory Medicine,
Thomayer University Hospital with Polyclinic, First Faculty of Medicine,
Charles University, Prague, Czech Republic

J. Rovensky et al. (eds.), *Sine Syndromes in Rheumatology*,
DOI 10.1007/978-3-7091-1541-1_10, © Springer-Verlag Wien 2014

develop erosive changes detectable on X-rays. The second case presents a patient with a serious pulmonary finding without significant articular involvement. Only the differential diagnostics of pulmonary findings and targeted examination of peripheral joints resulted in the diagnosis of rheumatoid arthritis.

Case Report No. 1: Absence of Erosive Changes on X-Rays in Spite of 20-Year Duration of Rheumatoid Arthritis

This case report presents a 63-year-old female patient with rheumatoid arthritis (RA) in whom the disease manifested with edema of ankles and MTP joints in 1990. Later the arthritic syndrome progressed with the involvement of knees, shoulders and small hand joints. At the onset of the disease, antimalarial agents (Delagil) were administered, followed by sulphasalazine (2 g/day) for 2 years. Sulphasalazine had to be discontinued due to hepatopathy. Later the patient temporarily took Plaquenil. In March, 2000, she started to take prednisone at 10 mg/day. In the period between March 2002 and September 2002 she took cyclosporine A that was replaced by leflunomide due to persisting activity of the disease.

In January 2003, a physical examination showed arthritic syndrome of PIP I, II, V on the right hand, MCP I bilaterally of the wrists and of the right knee with the presence of exudate and Baker's cyst in popliteal fossa, edema of ankles, painful crosswise pressure on MTP joints and atrophy of interosseal muscles. The patient complained of morning stiffness lasting for several hours.

Laboratory parameters were as follows: ESR: 82/105, HGB: 11.0 g/L, RBC: 4.170.000, WBC: 12.700, PLT: 471.000, urinalysis was negative, LFT: 24, HT: 56, ANA: negative.

X-rays showed the following findings: mild diffuse osteoporosis on hands, denser opacity of soft tissues in the right wrist, rhizarthrosis grade I on the left side; osteoporosis of feet, hallux valgus bilaterally, arthrosis of MTP I grade I on the right side, grade II on the left side; cervical spine: osteochondrosis of C4-7 discs grade II with anterior and posterior osteophytes, C3-4 osteochondrosis grade I, without the signs of atlantoaxial dislocation on dynamic X-rays; knees: diffuse osteoporosis, minimal narrowing of articular fissures bilaterally, tipping of intercondylar eminence bilaterally. Thermographic examination did not reveal the disorder of acral circulation suggesting Raynaud's phenomenon. Ultrasonography of the right knee revealed the presence of a small amount of thickened synovium up to 2 mm in suprapatellar recess with a minimal amount of fluid when applying pressure and reduction of cartilage of femoral condyles. A Baker's cyst was found in the popliteal fossa, consisting mostly of the tissue that was reaching up to the ankle joint along the medial side of the calf. An MRI scan of the wrists showed small effusions with synovial thickening in the left-sided metacarpal joint; similar changes could be seen in the ulnar part of the left wrist in close vicinity of os ipsiforme. Synovium was also mildly thickened in the area of metacarpophalangeal joints. Small articular effusion was found between the *os scaphoideum* and radius on the right side. Synovium thickening with the presence of small articular effusion was seen in the right-sided metacarpophalangeal joints, especially in MCP II and III. Discrete subchondral cystic changes of up to 4 mm were present in the proximal part of the radius head.

Conclusion: Described changes were typical for rheumatoid arthritis in the given localizations with accompanying synovium thickening and minimal articular effusion.

Diagnostic summary: This was a seropositive rheumatoid arthritis with polyarthritis, higher clinical and humoral activity. The disease began in 1990, with reactivation during the last 3 years. With regard to ineffective basal treatment with leflunomide, combined treatment with antimalarial agents and methotrexate after the wash-out phase with Questran was initiated in 2003.

Disease reactivation with high inflammatory activity occurred again in 2010, so the treatment with antimalarial agents was stopped and biologic therapy with tocilizumab was initiated. This treatment led to the regression of the arthritis and a decrease of acute phase reactants. In 2011, X-rays of the hands revealed subluxation and desaxation of carpometacarpal joint and metacarpophalangeal joint of right-sided first digit, bilateral finding of narrowing and even vanishing of articular fissure of the MCP joint of the second digit, more pronounced on the right side, bilateral small lateral osteophytes and subchondral sclerotization – stage 3, significant narrowing of RC joint space bilaterally with subchondral sclerotization. Feet: status post-resection of second to fourth metatarsus heads on the right side, arthrosis of MTP joint of big toe bilaterally, spindle-like widening in the middle part of the second metatarsus on the left side of a callus-like character.

Case Report No. 2: Rheumatoid Arthritis with Dominating Pulmonary Involvement and Oligosymptomatic Articular Involvement

The authors present the case of a 66-year-old female patient transferred to the Clinic of Pneumology of the 1st Medical School of Charles University, Thomayer's Teaching Hospital and Out-patient Clinic, Prague, due to a bilateral pulmonary process of unknown origin. Family history was negative regarding cardiovascular, pulmonary, malignant, rheumatologic and metabolic diseases. The patient had worked as a kindergarten teacher, and later on as a manual laborer at a printing house, and finally in a factory producing LP records. Currently she was retired. She lived in a family house and bred parrots. She smoked two cigarettes a day, and denied having allergies. Medical history was as follows: arterial hypertension, hyperlipidemia, type 2 diabetes on a diet and oral antidiabetics, hypothyroidism on the basis of chronic lymphocytic thyroiditis, cholecystolithiasis, hepatic steatosis and splenomegaly. The only surgery had been an appendectomy. She had been taking Lokren, Moduretic, Blessin, Euthyrox and Glucophage for a long time.

The patient was first examined at gastroenterology outpatient clinic in Beroun due to elevation of hepatic enzymes. To exclude a hepatic lesion, she was referred for an MRI scan of the liver. Lesion in the basal part of the right lung was described as a secondary finding. A chest CT scan was subsequently performed, with the finding of apparent bilateral large foci – cavities with thick walls. The patient was

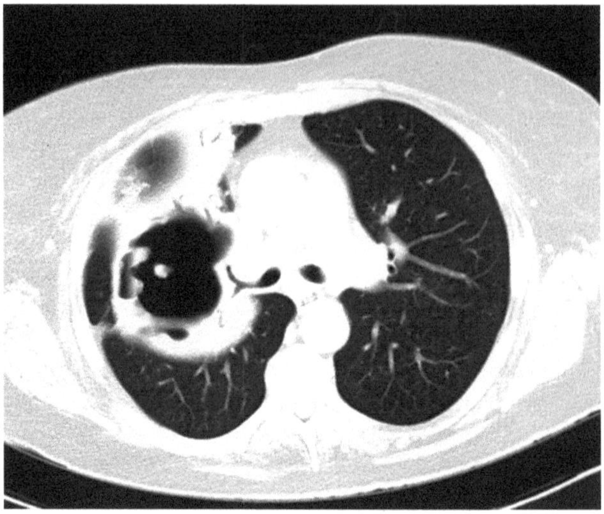

Fig. 1 Chest CT scan with the finding of secondarily infected decayed rheumatic node

hospitalized in the Department of Pneumology in Kladno Hospital. Bronchoscopies were repeatedly performed, with the finding of purulent secretion in bronchi with *Staphylococcus aureus* positivity in cultures; an *aspergillus* antigen blood test was also positive. A transparietal puncture of the focus under CT control did not prove to be of tumorous origin. The only interesting laboratory result was eosinophilia in peripheral blood. A quantiferon test was negative.

Physical examination at the time of admission: obesity, without dyspnea, blood pressure was 118/92 mmHg, O_2 saturation measured by pulse oxymeter was within the reference range (97 % without oxygenotherapy), normal respiratory sounds. Abdomen was over the chest level, without pathologic findings. Lower extremities were without edema or signs of phlebothrombosis. Signs of involvement of peripheral joints were not described.

Laboratory parameters were as follows: elevated IgE levels (711.8 IU/mL), only mildly elevated hepatic enzymes (AST 0.79 μkat/L, ALT 0.64 μkat/L, bilirubin 26.0 mmol/L, GMT 3.35 μkat/L), lower plasma albumin level (26.6 g/L), mild hyponatremia and hypokalemia (Na 133 mmol/L; K 3.2 mmol/L). On admission procalcitonin was also positive (1.82 ng/mL) as well as CRP (235.7 mg/L), glycemia was higher (9.70 mmol/L). Urinalysis was negative. Blood gases in peripheral arterial blood were within reference range. Blood count showed neutrophilia without left shift; eosinophil count was within reference range.

Repeated chest CT scans displayed multiple foci in both lungs – large cavity with wide level on the right side, probably corresponding to formed *aspergillus* cavities (Fig. 1). Bronchoscopic examination revealed considerably erythematous, edematous mucosa of bronchi with orifices from which yellow-green purulent secretions with a considerable putrescent odor was sucked off. Culture from bronchial lavage contained *Streptococcus viridans* and *Staphylococcus aureus* with preserved sensitivity to oxacillin. Mycological and mycobacteriologic tests were negative. On

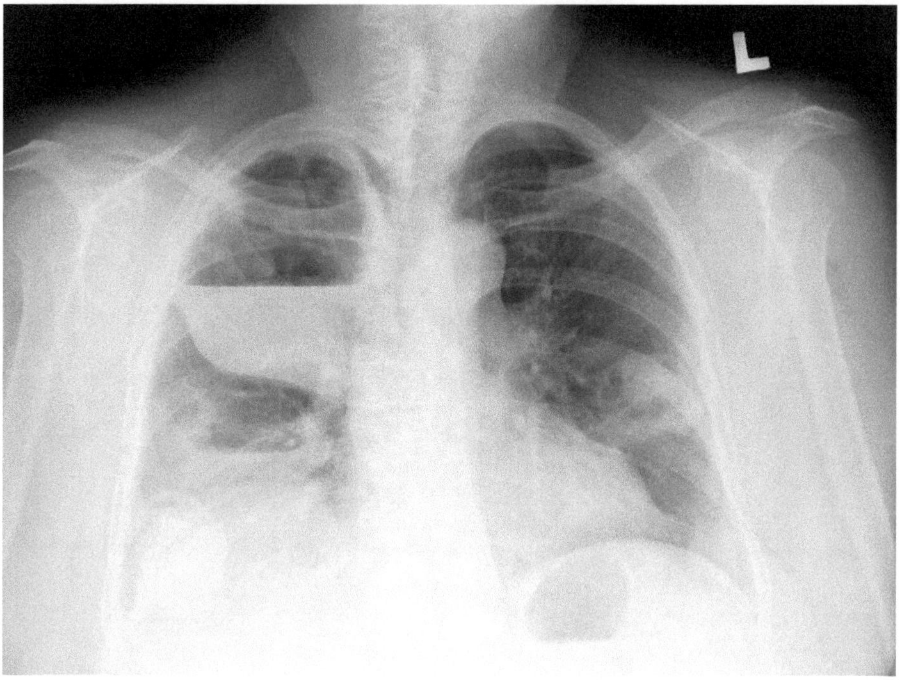

Fig. 2 Chest X-ray before antibiotic therapy

the basis of these results, we initiated combined antimicrobial treatment (ciprofloxacin, metronidazole, lincomycin). A follow-up bronchoscopic examination showed significant regression of purulent secretion, and extramural stenosis of the right upper bronchus and of the left main bronchus before the origin of the upper bronchus was found. According to macroscopic findings, it was assessed as suspected – inflammatory granulation. A biopsy of this granulation was examined histopathologically, finding sections of necrotic tissue detritus and organizing granulation tissues filled with intense mixed inflammatory cellularity with a high proportion of neutrophils and eosinophil granulocytes.

A follow-up chest X-ray after a week of antibiotic administration showed regression of the cavity size in the right upper lung field and reduction of hydroaeric phenomenon size at the inferior pole of the right hilus. Focus with decomposition in the right laterobasal part persisted. There was an apparent regression of round focus in the left lateral part, and another focus in the left middle field in the outer angle was unchanged (Figs. 2 and 3). As tumor and pulmonary mycosis were not confirmed, a systemic disease as the origin of multiple focal processes had to be excluded.

Skiagraphy of both hands was performed with the following findings: radiocarpal fissures were mildly narrowed, small erosions on os navicularis, more pronounced on the left side. Rhizarthrosis on the left hand. Apparent small erosions and usurations on the heads of MCP joints of third and fifth digits bilaterally, severe erosions and usurations on the head of the left MCP joint of the

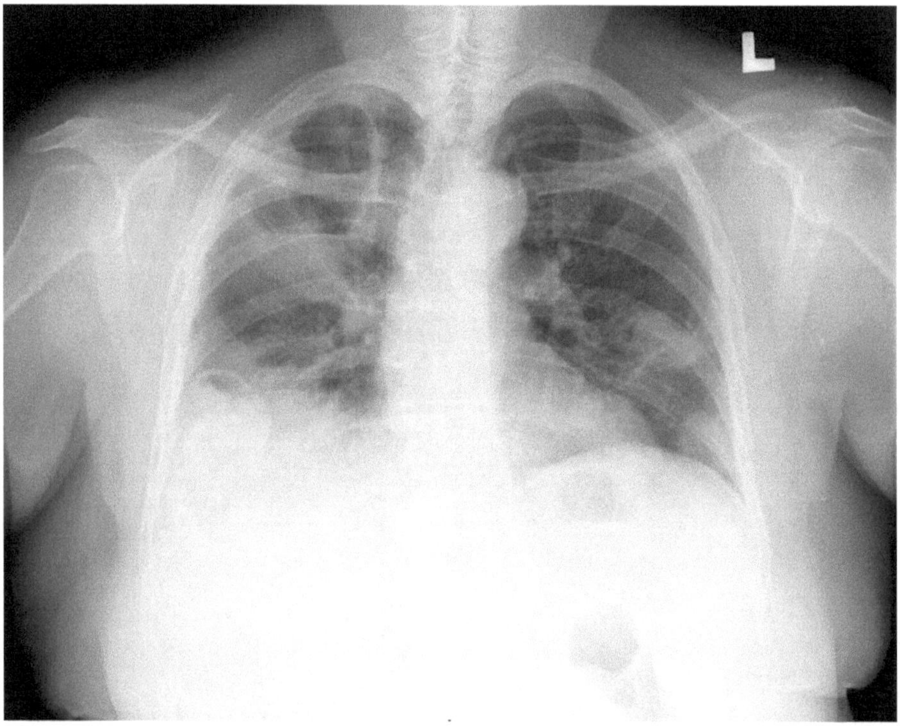

Fig. 3 Chest X-ray after antibiotic therapy

second digit, especially from the volar side, where there was a considerable subluxation position in a metacarpophalangeal joint, especially on the palmar side. Small erosions were also apparent on the bases of the digit phalanges. Cystoid translucency in the heads of MCP joints as well as digit phalanges. Mild narrowing of IP joints, some of them with minute tippings and with edema of soft tissues. Bouchard's node at the proximal IP joint of the fifth digit of the right hand.

Conclusion: The above-mentioned skeletal findings on the hand most probably correspond to the combination of arthritis signs with maximum involvement of the left metacarpophalangeal joint of the second digit with the combination of arthrotic changes.

Rheumatologic consultation was subsequently performed: the patient complained of joint problems lasting for about a year. She noticed deformities and lower muscle strength as well as mild edema of joints. After antibiotic therapy at the Department of Pneumology, joint edema regressed, but the joints did not bother her much. On examination: deformity of joints with ulnar deviation and atrophy of interosseal muscles were described on both hands and wrists. MCP and PIP joints were not painful on palpation, knees had arthrotic shape, other joints were normal.

Conclusion: Suspected rheumatoid arthritis stage II with erosions according to radiographic examination.

Immunological laboratory parameters showed positivity of anticitrulline antibodies (212.9) and anti-rheumatoid factor IgG antibodies (74.53) as well as cellular immunity disorder, probably secondary to infection. On the basis of the above-mentioned facts, the condition was assessed as rheumatoid arthritis with minimal articular symptoms and dominating pulmonary involvement with the formation of necrobiotic nodes with secondary infection. Rheumatic nodes were not found, other than in the pulmonary localization. After the hospital discharge we recommended continuingher with Biseptol administration to cure the superinfection and the patient was referred to regional rheumatology outpatient clinic.

Discussion

One of the important ACR classification criteria for the diagnosis of rheumatoid arthritis (RA) is the presence of X-ray changes typical for RA on postero-anterior skiagraph of the hand and wrist. The occurrence of RA without the development of X-ray changes is rare. In such cases, clinical findings usually change and after a couple of years a different nosologic entity can be recognized, namely from the group of diffuse connective tissue diseases, e.g., systemic lupus erythematosus (SLE). In SLE the arthropathy does not have the character of erosions.

In the first case, from the diagnostic point of view, there is no doubt that it is an active form of RA with considerable clinical and humoral activity. From the diagnostic criteria according to Arnett et al. [1] dated 1987, only the seventh of seven diagnostic criteria is not fulfilled regarding X-ray changes, because erosive changes were not demonstrated (X-rays assessed by two independent radiologist consultants). The open question is the cause of the absence of erosive changes on the hands and wrists.

Kirwan et al. [2] dealt with the problem of the administration of lower doses of prednisolone at an early stage of RA and they demonstrated that low dosages (7.5 mg daily) inhibited the development of erosive changes. Other literary sources confirm that low doses of corticosteroids (<10 mg/day) protect bone mass and significantly slow down the development and progression of erosions in RA [3–5]. Hickling et al. [6] similarly drew attention to the fact that prednisolone administration reduces the progression of erosive changes when comparing two groups of patients. The first group took classic therapy – DMARDs + prednisolone 7.5 mg daily, while the second took only DMARDs. The observed differences in the development of erosions after 2 years were in favor of the prednisolone group, in which erosion development was not demonstrated. However, the patients who discontinued prednisolone during the third year of therapy also developed erosive changes. The authors assume that low-dosage prednisolone administered at an early stage of the disease inhibits radiographic progression and its administration should be on a long-term basis.

The open issue is whether intermittent therapy with corticosteroids and various DMARDs had an impact on the inhibition of the development of erosive changes in our patient. This hypothesis requires further proof. Inflammatory processes within underlying disease, joint immobility, and increased vascularity around the joint dominantly participate in the development of localized bone loss in the form of periarticular osteopenia and bone erosions in RA [7]. The key role in bone mass reduction in RA is played by osteoclasts that can be directly activated by pro-inflammatory cytokines such as IL-1, TNF-α, IL-6 and a few others. Synovial tissue and chondrocytes also have the capability of producing various cytokines and growth factors (TNF, IL-1, IL-11, IL-17 and M-CSF) that can increase the formation, activity and survival of osteoclasts. Histological sections of a joint affected by arthritis demonstrate that multinuclear osteoclasts are present along the resorption lacunae in subchondral bone as well as at the areas of bone resorption on the border between bone and pannus [8].

Osteoclasts can also be activated via the essential mechanisms of the immune system, such as the receptor activator of nuclear factor κB – RANK and its ligand, RANKL (receptor activator of nuclear factor κB ligand). The RANKL antagonist is the soluble receptor protein called osteoprotegerin (OPG). OPG binds to RANKL and prevents its binding to RANK, thus inhibiting osteoclastogenesis, osteoclast function and, on the contrary, supporting their apoptosis [9]. In physiologic circumstances, osteoclastogenesis in the process of bone remodeling depends on the balance between RANKL-RANK and active OPG. In RA, RANKL is also expressed on activated T-lymphocytes (CD+T), on synovial fibroblasts and cartilage chondrocytes, which contributes to the disturbance of homeostasis between RANKL and OPG [10]. Hanyes et al. [11] demonstrated that OPG expression on synovial cells of the macrophage type as well as on endothelial cells is lacking in RA. On the contrary, RANKL expression in synovial tissue of the patients with active RA is higher when compared to patients with inactive RA, osteoarthrosis and controls [12]. Moreover, it has been demonstrated that the treatment of rats with OPG in adjuvant arthritis significantly reduces the number of osteoclasts and protects bone and joint structures [10]. The treatment of inflammatory bone loss in RA results from two principal requirements – reduction of bone resorption and increase of bone formation. New information on the development of periarticular osteoporosis and bone erosions in RA opens up new therapeutic options that besides basal treatment include anti-cytokine therapy, direct OPG application, inhibition of osteoclast function (bisphosphonates), activation of osteoblasts, etc. (Table 1). However, the patient primarily should receive efficient basal treatment that needs to exert anti-inflammatory properties and that has to slow down X-ray progression. In this context, methotrexate plays a historical role [13] and is successfully combined with sulphasalazine and antimalarial agents [14], cyclosporine A [15], in basal treatment.

The second case points out the diagnosis of RA that was determined on the basis of rheumatic nodules in lung tissue.

Pulmonary involvement in RA can be asymptomatic or it can be most commonly manifested by cough and dyspnea [16]. The case of a patient with multiple rheumatic nodules in the lungs and with pulmonary fibrosis leading to respiratory failure resulting in death is also described [17]. Rheumatic nodules occur in approximately 20 % of patients with RA. The incidence of rheumatic nodules in lung parenchyma occurs in about 1 % of the patients, while it is present in autopsy samples in 5 % of the

Table 1 Targeted strategies for the treatment of inflammatory bone loss in RA

Suppression of underlying pathological process, suppression of cellular immunity
Anti-cytokine therapy targeted on TNF, IL-1, IL-6, etc. Use of anti-inflammatory cytokines like IL-10, IL-13
Improvement of RANKL/OPG ratio in favor of OPG. Direct OPG application
Blocking osteoclast-bone interaction, inhibition of integrin receptor $\alpha v\beta 3$
Inhibition of osteoclast function (bisphosphonates)
Activation of osteoblast function (parathormone fragments)

Adapted from Rehman and Lane [10]

patients. They usually occur in those patients who also have subcutaneous rheumatic nodules and a positive serum rheumatoid factor. They are more often localized in the subpleural area in the right middle, or in both upper lung fields and they are more frequent in males. They are usually isolated, less frequently multiple, their size ranges from several millimeters to several centimeters. Nodules can become necrotic in the center where a cavity can be formed as well. After suppressing the disease activity, rheumatic nodules frequently regress and vanish [18, 19].

Rheumatic nodules usually occur in patients with the active, long-lasting form of RA. However, pulmonary nodules were also observed on HRCT scans in patients with early forms of RA [20]. In our patient, joint symptoms were searched for, only on the basis of an accidentally detected pulmonary ailment. A similar case was published by Voulgari et al. [21], who described asymptomatic solitary pulmonary nodules in a 54-year-old male patient who was a smoker. With regard to his age and smoking history, they were searching for a malignancy. Histological findings were characterized by numerous necroses with the rim of palisade-placed histiocytes and interstitial tissue with mononuclear cellular infiltrate as well as fibrosis. A similar histological finding was also detected in a subcutaneous nodule from the area of the right Achilles tendon, which was identical to the histological picture of the rheumatic nodule. A search through the medical history found arthralgia of the small hand joints that lasted for about 3 months and more than 1-h stiffness in the morning. The patient had elevated acute phase reactants and positivity of serum rheumatoid factor. On the basis of these findings, methotrexate therapy was initiated.

The asymptomatic occurrence of rheumatic nodules in lung parenchyma as the first symptom of RA is very rare. In these patients it is always necessary to exclude malignancies, tuberculosis, coincident granulomatosis with polyangiitis (Wegener's), fungal infections, and Caplan's syndrome [19, 21, 22].

References

1. Arnett FC, Edworthy SM, Bloch DA et al (1988) The American Rheumatism Association 1987 revised criteria for the classification of rheumatoid arthritis. Arthritis Rheum 31:315–324
2. Kirwan JR (1995) The effect of glucocorticoids on joint destruction in rheumatoid arthritis. N Engl J Med 333:142–146
3. Bjilsma JV, Van Everdingen AA, Huisman M et al (2002) Glucocorticoids in rheumatoid arthritis: effects on erosions and bone. Ann N Y Acad Sci 966:82–89

4. Lim SS, Conn DL (2001) The use of low-dose prednisolone in the treatment of rheumatoid arthritis. Bull Rheum Dis 50:1–4
5. Van Schaardenburg D, Valkema R, Dijkmans BAC et al (1995) Prednisone treatment of elderly onset rheumatoid arthritis. Disease activity and bone mass in comparison with chloroquine treatment. Arthritis Rheum 38:334–342
6. Hickling P, Jacoby RK, Kirwan JR (1998) Joint destruction after glucocorticoids are withdrawn in early rheumatoid arthritis. Arthritis and Rheumatism Council low dose glucocorticoid study group. Br J Rheumatol 37:930–936
7. Gravallese EM (2002) Bone destruction in arthritis. Ann Rheum Dis 61(Suppl 2):84–86
8. Suzuki Y, Nishikaku F, Nakatuka M, Koga Y (1998) Osteoclast-like cells in murine collagen induced arthritis. J Rheumatol 25:1154–1160
9. Lacey DL, Timms E, Tan HL et al (1998) Osteoprotegerin ligand is a cytokine that regulates osteoclast differentiation and activation. Cell 93:165–176
10. Rehman Q, Lane NE (2001) Bone loss. Therapeutic approaches for preventing bone loss in inflammatory arthritis. Arthritis Res 3:221–227
11. Haynes DR, Barg E, Crotti TN et al (2003) Osteoprotegerin expression in synovial tissue from patients with rheumatoid arthritis, spondyloarthropathies and osteoarthritis and normal controls. Rheumatology 42:123–134
12. Crotti TN, Smith ND, Weedon H et al (2002) Receptor activator NF-kappa B ligand (RANKL) expression in synovial tissue from patients with rheumatoid arthritis, spondyloarthropathy, osteoarthritis, and from normal patients: semiquantitative and quantitative analysis. Ann Rheum Dis 61:1047–1054
13. Pavelka K (1995) Současné postavení metotrexátu v léčbě revmatoidní artritídy. Čes Revmatol 3:16–23
14. O'Dell JR, Haire CE, Erikson N et al (1996) Treatment of rheumatoid arthritis with methotrexate alone, sulfasalazine and hydroxychloroquine or a combination of all three medications. N Engl J Med 334:1287–1291
15. Tugwell P, Pincus T, Yocum D et al (1995) Combination therapy with cyclosporin and methotrexate in severe rheumatoid arthritis. N Engl J Med 333:134–135
16. Kanat F, Levendoglu F, Teke T (2007) Radiological and functional assessment of pulmonary involvement in the rheumatoid arthritis patients. Rheumatol Int 27:459–466
17. Kitamura A, Matsuno T, Narita M et al (2004) Rheumatoid arthritis with diffuse pulmonary rheumatoid nodules. Pathol Int 54:798–802
18. Anwar A (2005) A review of pulmonary involvement in rheumatoid arthritis. APLAR J Rheumatol 8:16–18
19. Lukáč J, Lukáčová O (2010) Reumatoidná artritída. In: Lukáč J et al (eds) Systémové choroby spojivového tkaniva (systémové autoimunitné choroby). PN Print, s.r.o, Piešťany, pp S125–S151
20. Metafratzi ZM, Georgiadis AN, Ioannidou CV et al (2007) Pulmonary involvement in patients with early rheumatoid arthritis. Scand J Rheumatol 36:338–344
21. Voulgari PV, Tsifetaki N, Metafratzi ZM et al (2005) A single pulmonary rheumatoid nodule masquerading as malignancy. Clin Rheumatol 24:556–559
22. Hrnčíř Z, Toušek M (1962) Caplanův syndrom. Čas Lék Čes 101(27):850–853

Absence of Arthritis as a Sign of Sine Syndrome in Still's Disease in Adulthood

Jozef Rovenský, Veronika Vargová, Pavol Masaryk, and Elena Košková

Contents

Discussion 79
References 80

Abstract

The authors of this chapter discuss the atypical course of Still's disease in adulthood. It is a sine syndrome (skin changes, itchy, linear urticarial rash or other skin manifestations, periorbital edema and erythema of eyelids; organ manifestations were not present in the patient) with arthritis – in the form of monoarthritis of the right knee – that occurred after 23 years of the disease. The most pronounced feature was five attacks of fever associated with chills and high inflammatory activity. Therapy with corticosteroids, cyclosporine and methotrexate suppressed and reduced relapses of the disease. An attempt to discontinue basal therapy led to the last relapse of the disease. Differential diagnostic procedures for nosographic demarcation of Still's disease in adulthood associated with sine syndrome are discussed, as well as the options for future treatment with biologics.

J. Rovenský (✉)
National Institute of Rheumatic Diseases, Piešťany, Slovakia

Institute of Physiotherapy, Balneology and Therapeutic Rehabilitation, University of Saint Cyril and Methodius, Trnava, Piešťany, Slovakia
e-mail: jozef.rovensky@nurch.sk

V. Vargová
1st Department of Pediatrics and Adolescent Medicine, Faculty of Medicine, P. J. Šafárik University and University Children's Hospital, Košice, Slovakia

P. Masaryk • E. Košková
National Institute of Rheumatic Diseases, Nábrežie I. Krasku 4, Piešťany 921 12, Slovakia

J. Rovensky et al. (eds.), *Sine Syndromes in Rheumatology*,
DOI 10.1007/978-3-7091-1541-1_11, © Springer-Verlag Wien 2014

In 1897 George Frederic Still documented the form of chronic arthritis in children known as Still's disease, or "systemic onset of juvenile rheumatoid arthritis." According to the International League against Rheumatism (ILAR), we classify and call it a systemic form of juvenile idiopathic arthritis (sJIA). Juvenile idiopathic arthritis (JIA) includes all forms of arthritis that occur before age 16, persist for at least 6 weeks and whose etiology is unknown [1–4, 13]. One of the forms is systemic arthritis, which is the form that is associated and/or preceded by daily fever (1–2 peaks up to 39 °C a day for at least 2 weeks), and the presence of at least one of the following signs: volatile erythematous rash, generalized lymphadenopathy, hepatomegaly or splenomegaly and serositis [3, 4, 14]. The involvement of joints (arthritis) itself can occur several weeks or even years after the occurrence of the systemic signs [14]. A serious, potentially life-threatening form of systemic arthritis is the macrophage activation syndrome – MAS [2, 5].

Among the various names for RA in childhood, Grossman et al. [8] push JIA as the name for the whole nosologic entity, while Still's disease or syndrome are reserved for cases with a dominating triad of the signs – polyarthritis, lymphadenitis and splenomegaly. Wissler-Fanconi syndrome is a clinical variant of JIA, with the following signs: sepsis, high, usually intermittent fever, rheumatoid rash and leukocytosis present independently from preceding polyarthritis or associated with it [8]. Such a classification is generally not acknowledged and Still's syndrome has been used as the name for the whole set of signs, especially in recent years [1]. As the diagnosis of JIA (as well as Still's disease and syndrome respectively) is generally reserved for patients younger than 15 or 16 years respectively, it is basically not used when occurring in adults. Bywaters [2] mentioned the possibility of the occurrence of Still's syndrome and Wissler-Fanconi syndrome respectively in adult patients, and this observation was also confirmed by others [1, 5–7, 9, 11].

Arthritis does not have to be the principal clinical criterion for Still's disease in adulthood. In a multi-center trial comprising 65 patients, arthralgia without arthritis was present in 20 patients, of whom only three developed joint deformities [1]. Hajzok et al. [10] documented a group of six adult patients with Still's disease. Patient No. 1 developed arthritis 1 month after the onset of the disease, and patient No. 2 after 2 years. Patient No. 5 experienced acute onset with fever, carditis, and arthralgia with exanthema. Patient No. 6 first had volatile exanthema with fever that was followed by arthritis 2 weeks later, and patients Nos. 3 and 4 had arthritis present from the onset of the disease.

Although sJIA is defined as a disease of children with the onset before the age of 16, the course of the disease in adolescence can mimic the course in adults [12]. Prendiville et al. [12] documented in their paper five patients aged 11–15 with multi-organ inflammatory affliction, characteristic clinical findings such as fever, various forms of pruritus, and linear urticarial eruptions that were associated with febrile peaks, especially in the late afternoon and evening. All those patients had arthralgia and four of them had transient arthritis that did not develop into persistent articular disease in any of the patients. Other clinical symptoms included periorbital edema/erythema and non-linear urticarial lesions. Two children had splinter hemorrhages under their nail beds and one girl experienced a fixed squamous pigmented linear eruption. Apathy, myalgia, arthralgia and leukocytosis were documented in all patients. Other symptoms included sore throat, transient arthritis, abdominal pain, lymphadenopathy, hepatomegaly, splenomegaly, elevated ferritin levels, and hepatic dysfunction. Arthritis did not persist in any of the patients, and the course of the disease varied. Macrophage activation syndrome developed in one patient, who recovered after oral administration of Naproxen. Two patients responded well to systemic corticosteroid therapy. One girl experienced an epileptic seizure and then died from aspiration and asphyxia. Another boy developed severe hepatitis associated with renal failure and thrombotic thrombocytopenic purpura; he was treated with plasmapheresis, dialysis and systemic corticosteroid therapy. The patient had recurrent episodes of rash and fever until he reached adulthood.

These children did not fulfill the defined criteria of systemic idiopathic arthritis because persistent arthritis was not present. The adolescent and adult patients had the same clinical findings and laboratory parameters as described in Still's disease in adults. The recognition of various urticarial eruptions and febrile peaks is very important for the diagnosis of this disease, which can take a serious clinical course and be potentially life-threatening.

In our group of patients with sJIA, we describe the case of a 38-year-old male patient with disease onset at age 15 (1987). The administration of prednisone and plaquenil led to complete remission of the disease, but it was not possible to prevent recurrent attacks of the disease. Three attacks were documented until 1990, while polyarthritis did not occur during the recurrence. High fever with rash dominated the clinical findings; corticosteroids and methotrexate were used during the last attack (2001). The fourth attack occurred in April 2006. A peritonsillar abscess and minimal pericardial effusion were present during this attack, and arthritis was again absent. The patient recovered after pulse corticosteroid therapy and the addition of cyclosporine. Cyclosporine administration was continued. Corticosteroids were discontinued in the spring of 2010, but at the end of October 2010, a sudden relapse with sore throat and fever occurred that dominated the clinical findings. A physical examination did not reveal any other abnormalities, including arthritic syndrome. Laboratory parameters showed high ESR (93/125, 78/115) and high CRP levels (90, 90, 57 mg/L); protein electrophoresis was as follows: total proteins 62 g/L, alpha1-globulin 6.8 g/L, alpha2-globulins 13.2 g/L, betaglobulin 11.9 g/L, gammaglobulins 12 g/L. Anti-CCP and ANA antibodies were negative, RF was 14.8 IU/mL. Synoviogram was as follows: 30 mL of fluid, 22,000 nuclear cells. Echocardiographic findings were as follows: without dilatation and hypertrophy of heart cavities, preserved systolic and diastolic function, without vegetations, trace pericardial effusion behind the posterior wall of the left ventricle. Abdominal ultrasonography and CT scan revealed hepatosplenomegaly and liver hemangioma. Scintigraphy with labeled leukocytes documented signs of mild inflammatory infiltration in the area of the right knee, without pathologic findings in other areas.

Upon discharge, we wrote that he was a 38-year-old patient with a polycyclic form of Still's disease with the onset at age 15. The disease manifested with recurrent attacks, the last one in 2006. The patient continued with corticosteroids and cyclosporine until the spring of 2010 when therapy was discontinued due to remission. At the end of October 2010, a sudden relapse with sore throat and high fever occurred, but without exanthema. Antibiotics were initially administered; afterwards the patient was admitted to the local Department of Internal Medicine, where pulse corticosteroid therapy led to partial improvement of the condition. The patient was transferred to National Institute of Rheumatic Diseases Piešťany for further treatment. During the hospitalization we observed septic fever, high ESR and CRP, leukocytosis with the left shift (20 % of rods), and pseudopurulent exudate in the right knee; however, the culture was negative. *Staphylococcus aureus* was confirmed in one hemoculture, and the patient received antibiotics according to sensitivity results. Despite it, septic fever persisted. We performed a "leukoscint" examination that confirmed only low activity in the right knee. Similarly, procalcitonin levels were repeatedly slightly elevated, but not as in septic conditions. Echocardiography was negative as well as an ENT examination. Hyperechogenic focus in the liver as seen on ultrasonography was assessed as a hemangioma without dynamic changes; the finding was verified by a CT scan. We administered pulses of corticosteroids (Solu-Medrol 500 mg) with a short-term effect; therefore we adjusted the therapy to continual administration of higher doses (prednisone 60 mg/daily) with a gradual decrease. Body temperature stabilized, and ESR and CRP decreased slightly. Due to activation of arthritis in the left temporomandibular joint, we added methotrexate to the therapy. Nizoral was also added due to a yeast superinfection.

Case No. 2 is interesting from the point of view of differential diagnostics, previous course of the disease as well as future prognosis or availability of new therapeutic modalities.

We have been following a 19-year-old patient from the age of 2.5 when he first experienced fever of a "septic" character, associated with non-specific clinical findings with dominating generalized lymphadenopathy and hepatosplenomegaly. The elevation of non-specific inflammatory markers (ESR, CRP), anemia and leukocytosis with the prevalence of polymorphonuclear leukocytes dominated in laboratory parameters. We performed complete laboratory and imaging examinations from which we could not confirm infectious (viral, bacterial, fungal or parasitic) or malignant (hemoblastosis, lymphoma, neuroblastoma) etiology. Thus we determined the diagnosis of the systemic form of juvenile idiopathic arthritis "per exclusionem." We prescribed pulse methylprednisolone therapy (3 × 30 mg/kg/day), with the switch to prednisone at 2 mg/kg/day in combination with nonsteroidal anti-inflammatory drugs. This treatment had an excellent therapeutic effect; however, the reduction of the daily corticosteroid dosage below 0.25 mg/kg/day was associated with the recurrence of systemic signs. Despite the combination with available basal drugs (we successively added methotrexate, antimalarial drugs, sulphasalazine and cyclosporine A to the therapy), relapses of systemic manifestations appeared and the patient remained cortico-dependent. From 1996 until 2007 the disease recurred nine times. There was fever with chills, hepatosplenomegaly, transient myalgia and arthralgia, but still without arthritis or erythematous rash; does the patient, in hindsight, fulfill the diagnostic criteria of sJIA? Is it still "arthritis sine arthritis?" Except for two short periods of remission free of therapy (August 2006–December 2006 and July 2007–December 2007), the boy basically took corticosteroids during his entire childhood and adolescence. Even a maximum effort to prevent the adverse effects of long-term corticosteroid therapy could not stop the development of serious growth retardation with negative psychological impact, especially during adolescence. During the last relapse, in December 2007, the patient received the last pulse of methylprednisolone and he has been in clinical and laboratory remission without corticosteroid therapy since December 2010. What will the future course of his disease be? With regard to his age, we referred him to specialists for adults. Does the next relapse of systemic signs nowadays automatically have to mean returning to corticosteroid therapy?

Discussion

In patient No. 1 we confirmed sJIA sine arthritis in the period from 1987 until 2010, when monoarthritis of the right knee occurred. The course of the disease resembles the cases [12] that referred to the above-mentioned disease as adult-onset Still's disease, or systemic juvenile idiopathic arthritis sine arthritis. Our patient fulfilled the criteria of sJIA without arthritis for nearly 13 years, with monoarthritis of the right knee occurring in 2010. The disease's course was very atypical with regard to the fact that except for the high fevers with chills, there was a good therapeutic response to corticosteroid monotherapy and combined therapy with corticosteroids and methotrexate; a rash associated with itching was not present, but other cutaneous changes appeared. The patient did not experience abdominal pain, and lymphadenopathy was not present. This means that it is a sine syndrome of sJIA with the absence of cutaneous changes, arthritis and other organ manifestations, but with the presence of fever, high inflammatory activity (ESR, CRP, electrophoresis) and pseudopurulent synovial effusion. It has to be noted that the course of fever was similar to that in sJIA. In such conditions it is a big problem to carry out nosographic demarcation of the disease, and it is obligatory to rule out an infectious disease (no proof of infectious agent). The ineffectiveness of antibiotic treatment supports the assumption that high fever is associated with sJIA. It is also necessary to rule out malignant diseases and autoinflammatory diseases other than sJIA.

In patient No. 2, our opinion is that the diagnosis remains the same as we determined it at the onset of the disease – sJIA sine arthritis. In periods of remission, the patient was and still is free of clinical problems. Except for the above-mentioned adverse effects of long-term corticosteroid therapy, we have not confirmed by repeated examinations the development of organ complications as a possible sign of any other autoinflammatory disease.

Corticosteroids, immunosuppressive drugs, and nonsteroidal anti-inflammatory drugs have been used in the therapy of sJIA. Biologic therapy (anakinra and tocilizumab) has been recently used in sJIA. This kind of treatment can have better therapeutic results and fewer adverse effects as current treatment strategies in this relatively rare nosologic entity.

References

1. Bujak JS, Aptekar RG, Decker JL et al (1973) Juvenile rheumatoid arthritis in the adult as fever of unknown origin. Medicine (Baltimore) 52(5):431–444
2. Bywaters EGL (1971) Still's Disease in the adult. Ann Rheum Dis 30:121–131
3. Calabro JJ (1966) Juvenile rheumatoid arthritis. Arthritis Rheum 9(1):82–87
4. Calabro JJ, Marchesano JM (1968) Rash associated with juvenile rheumatoid arthritis. J Pediatr 72:811–819
5. Caroit M, Mathien M, Kahn ME et al (1973) Maladie de Still de l'adult et syndrome de Wissler-Fanconi. Rev Rhum 40(1):s1–s8
6. Cook PJ (1976) Adult Still's disease with late relapse. Proc R Soc Med 69(1):4
7. Davis GE, Fakhery B (1975) The unusual presentation of "Juvenile" rheumatoid arthritis in an adult. J Maine Med Assoc 66(3):78–80
8. Grossman BJ, Ozoa NE, Arya SC (1965) Problems in juvenile rheumatoid arthritis. Med Clin North Am 49(1):33–47
9. Gupta RC, Mills MD (1973) Still's disease in an adult: a link between juvenile and adult rheumatoid arthritis. Am J Med Sci 296(1):137–144
10. Hajzok O, Rovenský J, Lukáč J et al (1978) Klinický obraz Stillovej choroby v dospelom veku. Prakt Lek 58(1):20–24
11. Havelka S, Bardfeld R (1982) Polyarthritis progressiva juvenilie. Fysiat Věstn 40(3):157–165
12. Prendiville JS, Tucker LB, Cabral DA et al (2004) A pruritic linear urticarial rash, fever, and systemic inflammatory disease in five adolescents: adult-onset Still disease or systemic juvenile idiopathic arthritis sine arthritis? Pediatr Dermatol 21(5):580–588
13. Praken B, Albani S, Martini A (2011) Juvenile idiopathic arthritis. Lancet 377:2138–2149
14. Prince FH, Otten MH, van Suijlekom-Smit LW (2011) Diagnosis and management of juvenile idiopathic arthritis. Br Med J 342:95–102

Clinical Presentation of Sine Syndrome in Psoriatic Arthritis

Jozef Rovenský and Želmíra Macejová

Contents

Case Report ... 82
Discussion ... 83
References ... 85

Abstract

Sine syndrome occurs in approximately 20 % of psoriatic arthritis cases. From the clinical point of view, it is usually characterized by the presence of dactylitis and arthritis of DIP joints with the absence of skin involvement. HLA Cw6 tends to be present from genetic markers. In this case report, we describe the course of psoriatic arthritis sine psoriasis.

In 1973 Moll and Wright described psoriatic arthritis as a nosologic entity that often manifests with asymmetrical arthritis affecting DIP joints and joints of the anterior part of the chest [5]. Dactylitis, enthesitis, X-ray signs of bone formation, and the involvement of terminal phalanges also occur; extraarticular manifestations

J. Rovenský (✉)
National Institute of Rheumatic Diseases, Piešťany, Slovakia

Institute of Physiotherapy, Balneology and Therapeutic Rehabilitation, University of Saint Cyril and Methodius, Trnava, Piešťany, Slovakia
e-mail: jozef.rovensky@nurch.sk

Ž. Macejová
3rd Department of Internal Medicine, Faculty of Medicine, P. J. Šafárik University and L. Pasteur University Hospital, Košice, Slovakia

J. Rovensky et al. (eds.), *Sine Syndromes in Rheumatology*,
DOI 10.1007/978-3-7091-1541-1_12, © Springer-Verlag Wien 2014

(ophthalmic, cardiac) are typical. Scarpa et al. [13] propose the classification of psoriatic arthritis in three different forms from the point of view involvement:

1. Diagnosed psoriatic arthritis that manifests with apparent or regressing cutaneous changes or with nails affected by psoriasis.
2. Psoriatic arthritis sine psoriasis that occurs in patients without psoriasis, but the disease occurs in first- and second-degree relatives.
3. An early form of psoriatic arthritis that consists of joint involvement with recent onset that occurs in patients with evident forms typical for the diagnosis of psoriatic arthritis or in patients in the "sine psoriasis" group.

Psoriatic arthritis with sine syndrome occurs in approximately 20 % of all the patients with arthritis. From the clinical point of view, it is characterized by the presence of dactylitis and arthritis of DIP joints. The HLA Cw6 genetic marker is characteristic of sine syndrome in psoriatic arthritis. Clinical manifestation of a sine syndrome is characterized by joint involvement, but without apparent skin involvement. Scarpa et al. [10] point out the frequent occurrence of positive family history of psoriasis in first- and second-degree relatives. This means that on the basis of epidemiological studies, 20 % of the patients with sine syndrome in psoriatic arthritis have joint involvement that precedes the occurrence of skin involvement. In our case report, we present a disease course in a patient with sine syndrome in psoriatic arthritis.

Case Report

Patient: 48-year-old male

Past history: The patient has been treated for sarcoidosis since 1992. He took corticosteroids for 4–5 years. He has been followed for unstable hypertension since 1996 and treated for hyperuremic syndrome since 1997. He has been taking allopurinol for a long time.

Present complaint: Pain in small joints of hands and feet has been occurring since 1996. Later on, pain and edema of the wrists and knees appeared as well as pain in costochondral articulations. Fever and cutaneous changes were not present. Father's brother had a positive history of psoriasis. Patient's condition was assessed as seronegative arthritis; NSAIDs, combined with low dosages of corticosteroids, were added to the therapy.

In 2007 the patient was examined at National Institute of Rheumatic Diseases Piešťany. Laboratory parameters: moderate inflammatory activity, RF negativity, higher CRP values. HLA-typization confirmed the presence of HLA-A2, B18, 17 and Cw6 antigens. X-rays of the hands showed typical changes for stage II psoriasis (protuberance and erosions of styloid process of the right ulna and distal part of the left radius, of the right MCP 2–4, left MCP 3–5, PIP 3 bilaterally and left DIP 2). With regard to clinical presentation, typical X-ray findings, family history, presence of HLA-B17 and Cw6 antigens and negativity of rheumatoid factor, the condition was assessed as psoriatic arthritis stage II sine psoriasis. The patient started to take NSAID, DMARDs (sulphasalazine) and had local cryotherapy on affected joints. Despite this treatment, the disease still progressed, markers of inflammation repeatedly increased, and polyarthritic syndrome persisted. Methotrexate was added to the therapy in 2009. Despite this therapy modification, we did not succeed in inducing remission; polyarthritis persisted as well as higher humoral activity (ESR: 32/h, CRP: 25 mg/L). In February 2011, clinical activity assessed by DAS28 index was 6.99 (number of painful joints: 20, number of swollen joints: 12, total patient's VAS: 78, ESR: 32/h). The patient was referred for anti-TNF therapy (etanercept), which led to a decrease in inflammatory activity; ESR and CRP levels reached reference range after 3 months of therapy: ESR: 10/h, CRP: 4.10. DAS28 score decreased to 2.68. In the course of the therapy, hepatic enzymes became elevated and therefore it was inevitable that the methotrexate had to be discontinued. Currently the patient takes sulphasalazine, an NSAID (Flugalin), and etanercept. His condition is clinically stable; the DAS28 score was 2.34 in January 2012. Markers for inflammation and hepatic enzymes were not elevated during laboratory check-ups.

Discussion

Psoriatic arthritis belongs to the class of diseases that affect musculoskeletal and skin structures. Cutaneous changes and nail affection usually precede or occur simultaneously with rheumatologic symptoms. In psoriatic arthritis, rheumatologic manifestations precede the occurrence of skin lesions in approximately 20 % of the patients [3, 12]. If there is a positive family history of psoriasis, we can speak about psoriatic arthritis sine psoriasis [6, 10]. In 2009, Olivieri et al. [7] carried out the study of a continual follow-up of 78 patients with an early form of psoriatic arthritis, of whom 13 (17 %) had psoriatic arthritis sine psoriasis. Olivieri et al. [7] state that in the past, psoriatic arthritis sine psoriasis was diagnosed in patients who had undifferentiated spondylarthritis. The clinical spectrum of patients with undifferentiated spondylarthritis includes incomplete forms of spondylarthritis (e.g., reactive spondylarthritis with the presence of asymptomatic infection and PsA sine psoriasis or an early form of spondylitis in a pre-radiographic stage of ankylosing spondylitis, while the above-mentioned form remains undifferentiated for a long time) [8].

Olivieri et al. [6] followed the patients with PsA for 12 months and they focused on clinical spectrum of symptoms of PsA. Inclusion criteria consisted of clinical symptoms and signs suggesting PsA and psoriasis in first-degree relatives in the absence of other rheumatic disease. Sixteen females and four males were examined. The average age of the 20 patients was 44.1 (15–77), and the mean duration of the disease was 5.3 (1–30) years. From the point of clinical manifestation, five patients had peripheral arthritis, peripheral tendosynovitis and tendosynovitis, two had peripheral arthritis and tendosynovitis, four had peripheral enthesitis and tendosynovitis, one had peripheral arthritis and peripheral enthesitis, three had only peripheral arthritis and one patient had only peripheral enthesitis; 15 patients fulfilled Amor's criteria [1]. These were 11 criteria of the European working group for spondylarthritis criteria and ESSG criteria [2]. Results of the study showed that the clinical spectrum of PsA sine psoriasis seems to be broad, and that sensitivity for PsA sine psoriasis is missing in Amor's and ESSG criteria.

Scarpa et al. [10] recently published the study that dealt with clinical presentations and genetic aspects of PsA sine psoriasis. The group included 57 patients

(31 females and 26 males) with undifferentiated spondylarthritis during 9 months of follow-up. Clinical analysis showed that dactylitis and arthritis in distal interphalangeal joints occurred unequivocally more frequently in patients with a positive family history of psoriasis. The presence of the HLA Cw6 antigen was significantly more frequent in patients with a positive psoriasis history than with a negative one. On the basis of HLA-typization, it was demonstrated that the B-27 antigen was significantly more frequent if the family history of psoriasis was negative. The presence of HLA-Cw6 was associated with DIP arthritis and dactylitis. The conclusion of the study states that the occurrence of PsA sine psoriasis as a nosologic sub-entity is identified by dactylitis and/or DIP arthritis, HLA-Cw6 presence and a positive family history of psoriasis.

Two forms of psoriasis vulgaris exist: hereditary, with the onset between the ages of 15 and 25, and sporadic, which has a later onset [4]. Rahman et al. [9] pointed out that 80 % of the patients with early onset have the positivity of HLA-Cw6, and a strong family history associated with the occurrence of skin lesions and development of arthritis. The patients with sine syndrome in PsA have a broad-spectrum history. The clinical presentation is characterized by dactylitis and/or DIP arthritis, the presence of the HLA-Cw6 antigen, and a positive family history of psoriasis. The classification criteria for psoriatic arthritis (CASPAR) allow the classification of psoriatic arthritis sine psoriasis [16].

The problems of PsA sine psoriasis or nail lesion were documented by Taniguchi and Kamatani in 2007 [14]. The authors presented the clinical course of the disease in a patient with classical features of PsA without the occurrence of psoriasis or nail lesions for 21 years; this was a 38-year-old male who experienced polyarthralgia in 1985. The patient did not have any health problems other than diffuse edema of the big toe that lasted for 1 month. During the 19 years of follow-up, the patient experienced asymmetrical polyarthritis, primarily on the hands and feet, including DIP joints. During the clinical follow-up, dactylitis of the fingers and big toe as well as enthesitis that affected insertion of Achilles tendon and insertion of quadriceps muscle on patella occurred. Sacroiliac joints or spine were not affected. Subcutaneous lesions, psoriasis or nail affection were not observed. Laboratory parameters showed higher levels of red blood cells and CRP. Antinuclear antibodies were not present, the rheumatoid factor was negative, and antibodies against *Chlamydia trachomatis* were absent. X-rays of the hands and feet showed a tendency to the destruction of DIP joints with irregular distribution. Large ankyloses in IP joints of the hands and feet associated with bone proliferation were also observed. Periostitis was present on finger phalanges. Arthritis distribution was asymmetrical, which was demonstrated by scintigraphic (99mTc) examination. The disease was resistant to therapy with gold salts and sulphasalazine; methotrexate was discontinued due to adverse effects and persistent arthritis on hands and feet. Partial effect was achieved with minocycline therapy.

In other papers published by Scarpa et al. [11], it was demonstrated that in 47 consecutively followed patients with early forms of PsA, 29 had a definitive form of PsA and 18 had a sine psoriasis form. An early form of PsA had an oligo-enthesoarthritic pattern in 75 % of the studied patients. Bone scintigraphy was increased three times when compared to clinical findings ($p<0.001$). Joint ultrasonography confirmed inflammation of the synovial membrane and/or tendons in all active areas of bone scintigraphy, but clinical examination of the patients was negative. The presence of articular and tendon erosions detected by standard X-ray methods was found in seven patients.

Finally, Taniguchi et al. [15] presented the case of a 57-year-old female with polyarthritis since 2008. The patient's medical history included arthritis of the knee joints and dactylitis, but cutaneous changes that would suggest psoriasis never occurred. A family history of psoriasis was also negative. Clinical findings included musculoskeletal manifestations of PsA with peripheral arthritis, axial involvement, enthesitis and dactylitis. The disease course suggested that significant destructive disease dominated in PsA sine psoriasis, while arthritis of the knee joints went into remission. Laboratory parameters were as follows: elevated alkaline phosphatase, CTx and NTx levels. The authors pointed out that elevated markers of bone resorption could precede PsA with the occurrence of severe bone-joint destructions.

References

1. Amor B, Dougados M, Mijiyawa M (1990) Criteria of the classification of spondylarthropathies. Rev Rhum Mal Osteoartic 57:85–89
2. Dougados M, van der Linden S, Juhlin R et al (1991) The European Spondylarthropathy Study Group preliminary criteria for the classification of spondylarthropathy. Arthritis Rheum 34:1218–1227
3. Gladman DD, Rahman P, Krueger GG et al (2008) Clinical and genetic registries in psoriatic disease. J Rheumatol 35:1458–1463
4. Henseler T, Christophers E (1985) Psoriasis of early and late onset: characterization of two types of psoriasis vulgaris. J Am Acad Dermatol 13:450–456
5. Moll JM, Wright V (1973) Psoriatic arthritis. Semin Arthritis Rheum 3(1):55–78
6. Olivieri I, Ciancio G, Padula A et al (2000) Psoriatic arthritis sine psoriasis: a study of 20 consecutive patients [abstract]. Arthritis Rheum 43(Suppl):S105
7. Olivieri I, Padula A, D'Angelo S et al (2009) Psoriatic arthritis sine psoriasis. J Rheumatol 36(Suppl 83):28–29
8. Olivieri I, van Tubergen A, Salvarani C et al (2002) Seronegative spondyloarthritides. Best Pract Res Clin Rheumatol 16:723–739
9. Rahman P, Schentag CT, Gladman DD (1999) Immunogenetic profile of patients with psoriatic arthritis varies according to the onset of psoriasis. Arthritis Rheum 42:822–823
10. Scarpa R, Cosentini E, Manguso F et al (2003) Clinical and genetic aspects of psoriatic arthritis "sine psoriasis". J Rheumatol 30:2638–2640
11. Scarpa R, Cuocolo A, Peluso R et al (2008) Early psoriatic arthritis: the clinical spectrum. J Rheumatol 34:137–141
12. Scarpa R, Oriente P, Pucino A et al (1984) Psoriatic arthritis in psoriatic patients. Br J Rheumatol 23:246–250
13. Scarpa R, Peluso R, Atteno M (2007) Clinical presentation of psoriatic arthritis. Rheumatismo 59(Suppl 1):49–51
14. Taniguchi A, Kamatani N (2007) A case of psoriatic arthritis without the appearance of psoriatic skin or nail lesions for 21 years. J Rheumatol 10:306–309
15. Taniguchi Y, Kumon Y, Shimamura Y et al (2011) Rapidly progressive destructive arthritis in psoriatic arthritis sine psoriasis: do bone resorption marker levels predict outcome of bone destruction in psoriatic arthritis? Mod Rheumatol 21(1):106–108
16. Taylor W, Gladman D, Helliwell P et al (2006) Classification criteria for psoriatic arthritis: development of new criteria from a large international study. Arthritis Rheum 54:2665–2673

Sine Syndromes in Ankylosing Spondylitis

Jiří Štolfa

Contents

Case Report No. 1 89
Discussion 90
Case Report No.2 92
Discussion 92
References 94

Abstract

The diagnosis of ankylosing spondylitis is currently based on the proof of sacroiliitis on X-rays. Therefore the term of "ankylosing spondylitis without sacroiliitis" might seem illogical. However, the clinical course of ankylosing spondylitis is (like in other rheumatic inflammatory diseases) highly variable, ranging from mild asymptomatic forms to rapidly progressive ones resulting in ankylosis of the spine or replacement of hip joints, in rhizomelic forms or even in extra-articular manifestations. Thus ankylosing spondylitis can be well "hidden" in this broad spectrum of clinical manifestations. A new concept of axial (and peripheral) spondyloarthritis throws some other light on these issues, which can explain these forms as so-called "pre-radiographic stage of axial spondyloarthritis."

The term of "ankylosing spondylitis without sacroiliitis" undoubtedly belongs to "sine syndromes" since the diagnosis is based on diagnostic criteria where the principal criterion defining the disease is missing, i.e. sacroiliitis in this case. As to the most currently valid and commonly used modified New York criteria dated 1984, low back pain and stiffness more than 3 months, improving with exercise, but not

J. Štolfa
Institute of Rheumatology, Prague, Czech Republic
e-mail: stol@revma.cz

J. Rovensky et al. (eds.), *Sine Syndromes in Rheumatology*,
DOI 10.1007/978-3-7091-1541-1_13, © Springer-Verlag Wien 2014

relieving by rest; limitation of lumbar spine motion in sagittal and frontal planes; chest expansion decreased relative to normal values for age and sex such a situation should not occur since the inevitable prerequisite for the definitive diagnosis of ankylosing spondylitis is just X-ray demonstration of sacroiliitis (sacroiliitis grade II bilaterally or grade III unilaterally) and one of clinical criteria [1]. From this point of view, it will be necessary to look at the diagnosis of ankylosing spondylitis from a more complex prospective while taking into account new insights into this disease.

The diagnosis of ankylosing spondylitis (AS) was historically based on X-ray demonstration of sacroiliitis [2]. This concept was confirmed by other authors and thus X-ray signs of sacroiliitis became the decisive criterion for establishing the diagnosis of AS.

In the 1970s British authors Moll and Wright created the concept of "seronegative spondyloarthritis" as a group of inflammatory diseases of the locomotor system that differed from rheumatoid arthritis (seronegativity and absence of rheumatic nodes), and were characterized by similar clinical manifestations, such as inflammatory affection of the axial skeleton (sacroiliitis or spondylitis) and affection of peripheral joints, skin and mucous membranes. Besides AS, they included psoriatic arthritis, reactive arthritis and arthritis associated with inflammatory bowel disease (ulcerative colitis and Crohn's disease) into this group [3]. Later, Behcet's disease and Whipple's disease were excluded from this group. This concept was also supported by the discovery (1973) of a strong association between the HLA B27 antigen and ankylosing spondylitis (80–95 %) and to a lesser extent with the other diseases in this group.

In the 1990s this group of diseases was extended by a special group of "undifferentiated spondyloarthritis" as a reaction to the fact that the disease had typical features of the group in many patients, but did not fulfill the diagnostic criteria of any of the above-mentioned clinical entities (Amor's criteria of spondyloarthritis and ESSG [European Spondylarthropathy Study Group] criteria) [4, 5]. The first diagnostic criteria of ankylosing spondylitis were detailed in 1961 – "Rome criteria" [6]. As the only criteria, they allow the diagnosis of AS without X-ray signs of sacroiliitis since the definitive diagnosis of AS can be made either in the presence of bilateral X-ray sacroiliitis and one or more clinical criteria, or only in the presence of four out of five clinical criteria (inflammatory pain in the lower back, pain and stiffness in the thoracic spine, limited movement in the lumbar spine, limited chest expansion and current or previous iritis or its consequences). New York criteria dated 1966 [7] excluded pain in the thoracic spine (due to low specificity) and iritis (due to low sensitivity) from the criteria; however, they require the presence of X-ray sacroiliitis for the definitive diagnosis of AS, as well as their last modification, dated 1984 (modified New York criteria) [1]. These modified criteria require the fulfillment of the X-ray criterion (sacroiliitis grade II bilaterally or grade III unilaterally) and the presence of one clinical criterion (inflammatory back pain, limited movement of lumbar spine in two planes, limited chest expansion with respect to age and gender) for the diagnosis of AS.

It is known that the interval between the onset of problems and diagnosis of AS is long and ranges from 6 to 8 years [8]. In a cross-sectional study in Middle- and East-European populations, it was 6–7 years [9]. The reason is the late X-ray manifestation of sacroiliitis. The situation changed after the implementation of magnetic

Table 1 Characteristic features of spondyloarthritis

Inflammatory back pain
Arthritis
Enthesitis (heels)
Uveitis
Dactylitis
Psoriasis
Crohn's disease/ulcerative colitis
Good response to non-steroidal anti-inflammatory drugs
Presence of spondyloarthritis in relatives
HLA B27 positivity
Elevated C-reactive protein (CRP)

resonance imaging (MRI) into the diagnostics of sacroiliitis. MRI is capable of visualizing the presence of inflammation in the area of sacroiliac joints even when destruction of articular areas is not yet present and only bone marrow edema (BME) can be observed. It was proved that active sacroiliitis on MRI scans (BME) predicts later development of "X-ray" sacroiliitis [10, 11]. This enables establishing the diagnosis of AS at an early, i.e., pre-radiographic stage. In spite of the fact that the majority of patients with the finding of acute sacroiliitis on MRI develop classical ("radiographic") ankylosing spondylitis, this is not true in all cases and some of the patients can remain in this stage without developing classical AS, which can result in diagnostic uncertainties. This (as well as other reasons), led to the concept of "axial spondyloarthritis" which includes these "pre-radiographic stages" as well as the conditions where a patient has clinical features of spondyloarthritis but he/she does not have sacroiliitis, which would best correspond to the term of "ankylosing spondylitis without sacroiliitis".

Axial spondyloarthritis (AxSpA) can be diagnosed in patients with chronic back pain (lasting ≥ 3 months) and manifesting before the age of 45, in two ways: (1) by "X-ray" criterion, i.e., active sacroiliitis on MRI or definitive sacroiliitis on X-rays according to modified New York criteria + ≥1 characteristic features of spondyloarthritis (Table 1) or (2) by clinical criterion, i.e., the presence of HLA B27 antigen + ≥ 2 characteristic features of spondyloarthritis, i.e. also without the presence of sacroiliitis [12].

The term "ankylosing spondylitis without sacroiliitis" can include the following conditions:

1. *Pre-radiographic stage of AS.* Patients in this stage of the disease can have the same urgent symptoms as patients with the definitive (radiographic) form of the disease and they can require the same therapy, i.e., NSAIDs, and in case of inadequate response, also biological therapy (anti-TNFα).

Case Report No. 1

The patient: T.K., 32 years old. Family history: insignificant. Personal history: arterial hypertension, on medication, otherwise insignificant. He works as a manager, smokes 15 cigarettes/day.

Current disease began relatively suddenly and presented with pain in the left hip joint since November 2010. The next month pain in the right hip joint occurred as well. Pain was first manifested only on exertion, later also at rest and during the night. The patient also complained of mild inflammatory pain of the lower back. A more detailed examination was performed in February 2011. Laboratory parameters showed mildly elevated C-reactive protein (CRP) and positive HLA B27 antigen. A clinical examination revealed painful movement limitation of both hip joints in all directions and shortened distances of the lumbar spine (Schober's distance, lateroflexion); peripheral arthritis was not present. Skeleton scintigraphy documented intense accumulation of radionuclide in both hip joints (more accentuated on the right side), mild accumulation in both shoulder joints, in sternoclavicular, costochondral articulations and in the area of the xiphoid process. X-rays documented aseptic necrosis bilaterally – Fig. 1a, b. X-ray of sacroiliac joints was normal; later the absence of sacroiliitis was also confirmed by negative findings on an MRI. Arthritis of MCP, PIP and wrist joints was temporarily present in February 2011. X-ray as well as clinical findings in hips progressed and required replacement of both hip joints (the right one in November 2011 and the left in July 2012). After both operations the patient feels well; minimal inflammatory pain of the lower back persists as well as stable mild distance shortening of the lumbar spine. CRP values returned to normal. He requires administration of non-steroidal anti-inflammatory drugs (NSAIDs) only seldom.

Discussion

The diagnosis of the patient can be formulated in different ways: (1) Like AS grade I (the patient had been diagnosed with this at a different clinic) – he had corresponding clinical symptoms: inflammatory back pain and shortened distances, but without the X-ray sacroiliitis that was also ruled out by MRI scans later. The disease manifested with hip pain and limited movement and the condition was assessed as a "rhizomelic" form of AS. However, the cause of coxalgia was rapidly progressive osteonecrosis of the femur head on X-rays – first on the right side and later on the left – requiring replacement of both hip joints. Rhizomelic involvement in AS is a relatively frequent manifestation, especially in young patients, and in such cases it represents a significant predictor of a severe course of AS in the future. Nevertheless, the principal disease in this patient had a mild course until now (only slight CRP elevation, mild back pain without X-ray changes); moreover, septic necrosis of the femur head is not a typical manifestation of AS. The involvement of hip joints in this patient is probably not associated with the underlying disease, despite the fact that a different cause could not be identified. Therefore we can (currently) conclude that it is "idiopathic" osteonecrosis, so the diagnosis of ankylosing spondylitis is uncertain. (2) This disease can be best characterized by the diagnosis of axial spondyloarthritis. The "clinical branch" of the diagnostic algorithm (HLA B27 presence + two of characteristic features of SpA – Table 1) enables making the diagnosis also without the presence of sacroiliitis. Except for the presence of the HLA B27 antigen, this patient has inflammatory back pain, arthritis observed by a physician in the past, and elevated CRP. At the same time, this diagnosis does not exclude developing into another defined disease from the spondyloarthritis group in the future.

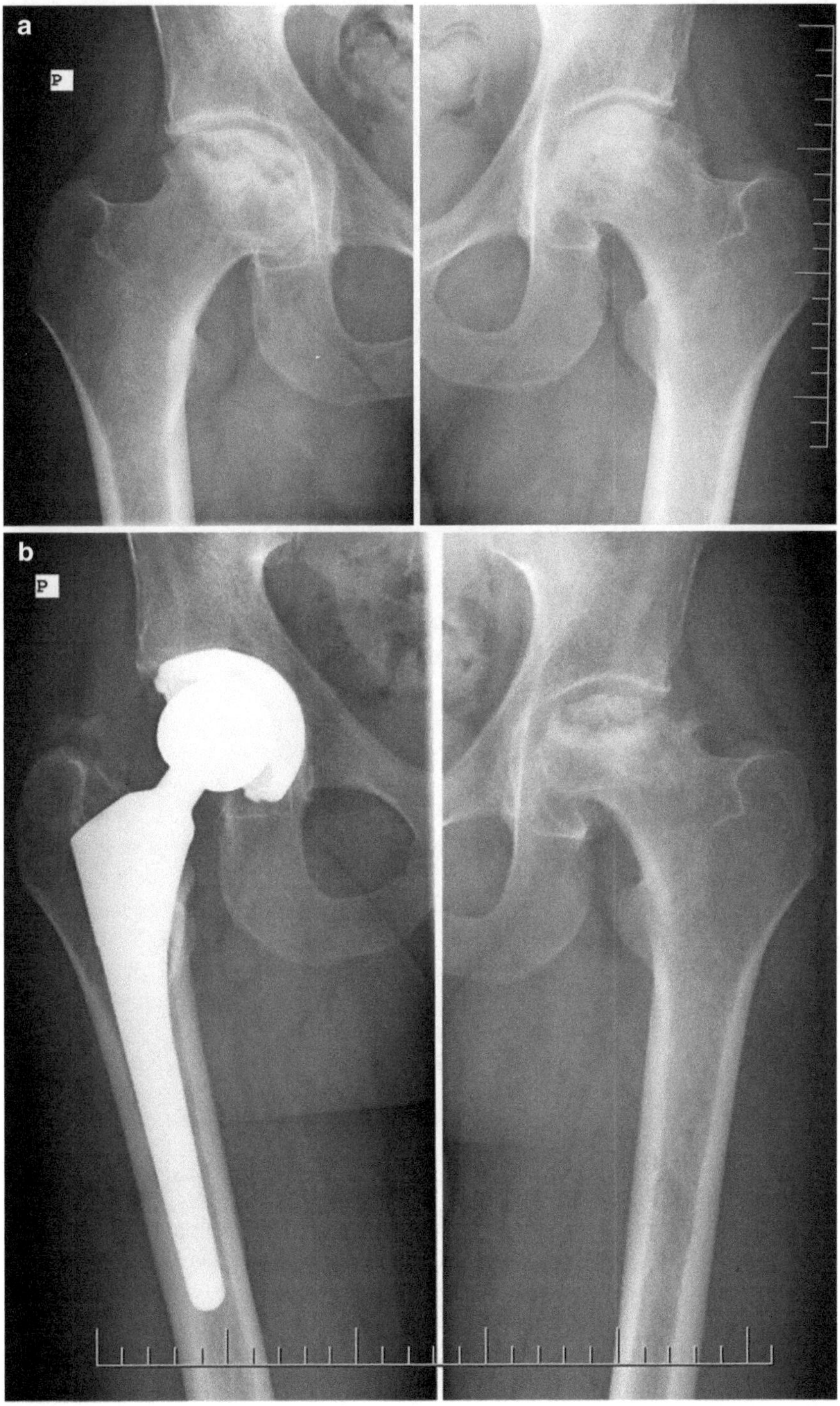

Fig. 1 (**a**) X-ray of hip joints dated November 2011: Severe osteonecrosis of head of the right hip joint and incipient necrosis on the left side. (**b**) X-ray of hip joints dated November 2012: Hip joint prosthesis on the right side, significant progression of osteonecrosis of head of the left hip joint when compared to X-rays dated 2011

2. *Ankylosing spondylitis in women.* Axial involvement in women with spondyloarthritis is less common than in men. While in classic AS (i.e., "radiographic" form of spondyloarthritis) the incidence ratio in men to women is 3:1; in AS without sacroiliitis (pre-radiographic or non-radiographic form of SpA) it is the same (1:1) [13–15]. The disease course is usually milder, and can also be manifested with isolated pain of the cervical spine, without problems in the lumbar area [16, 17]. Women also have more frequent involvement of peripheral joints [18] and more frequent uveitis during pregnancy [19]. The disease in women is more commonly accompanied by depression.
3. *Descendent forms of AS* are also more common in women. The first manifestation of the disease can be painful stiffness of the neck [16]. Sacroiliitis can be manifested later
4. *Axial form of other diseases from spondyloarthritis group,* where sacroiliitis is not a prerequisite for the diagnosis of the axial form (typically in psoriatic arthritis – PsA). It probably depends on the positivity of the HLA B27 antigen that is more common in patients with the disease manifesting at a young age and with axial involvement, and less common in patients with the disease manifesting at a later age, with more frequent peripheral involvement (it is typically reactive or psoriatic arthritis with HLA B27 positivity in 20–70 % patients) [20]. Inflammatory back pain without demonstration of corresponding X-ray changes was also seen in Crohn's disease [21].

Case Report No.2

A 58-year-old patient with inflammatory back pain since 1995, with shortened distances in the lumbar and thoracic spine, with the manifestation of polyarthritis in 1998. He has suffered from psoriasis since 1991 (type I with the manifestation before age 40, with a positive family history of psoriasis – father suffered from it as well). During the follow-up, markers of inflammation (ESR, CRP) were within the reference range; HLA B27 antigen was negative. Spine X-rays showed marked parasyndesmophytes – Fig. 2a, b; there were normal findings on sacroiliac joints, without signs of sacroiliitis. Peripheral joints: small destructive changes in DIP joints in upper extremities and in MTP joints in lower extremities.

Discussion

Inflammatory back pain, shortened distances and X-ray findings on thoracic-lumbar margin and on lumbar spine undoubtedly suggested spondyloarthritis in this patient, but it would also be possible to consider ankylosing spondylitis in the differential diagnostic process. The absence of sacroiliitis and special shape of osteophytes in the spine of a parasyndesmophyte character led to the consideration of another type of spondyloarthritis in the presence of psoriasis – an axial form of psoriatic arthritis – PsA (the patient has also involvement of the peripheral joints).

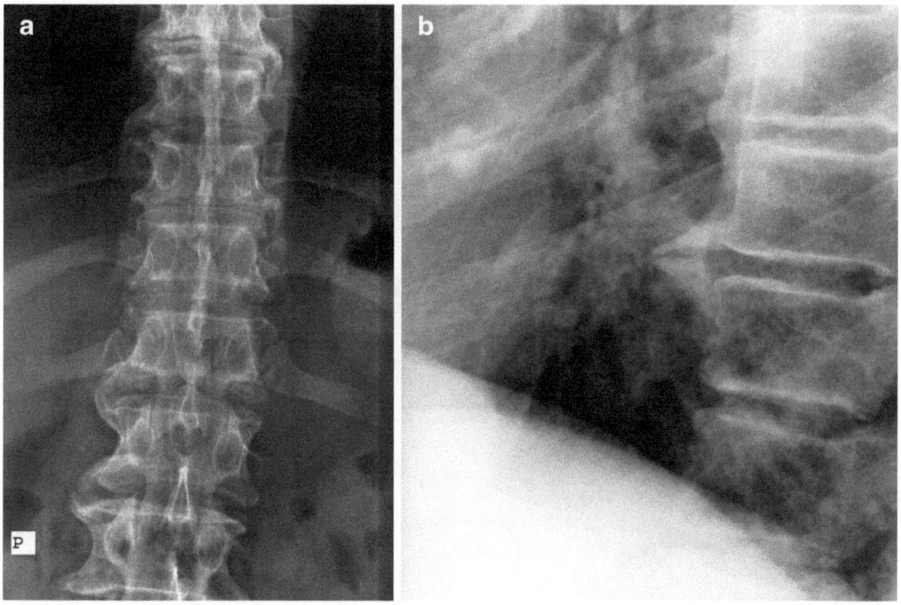

Fig. 2 (**a**) Hyperostotic formations on vertebral bodies in nearly all segments, ventrally as well as laterally; some of them have the character of bull horns. At Th12/L1 level they have abridging character laterally on the right side (**b**)

It is "spondyloarthritis without sacroiliitis," an axial involvement common in PsA. This usually does not cause major problems, is not associated with the elevation of acute phase reactants, and generally does not progress significantly.

5. *Atypical forms of ankylosing spondylitis.* The following asymptomatic forms of the disease can be included here:
   (a) Asymptomatic course and characteristic X-ray signs, i.e., mild forms of the disease. Their incidence in the literature ranges from 1.5 to 10 % [22].
   (b) Asymptomatic course with dominating extra-articular manifestations.
   (c) Symptomatic course without corresponding X-ray signs (i.e., without sacroiliitis).

While taking into account the still valid classification criteria, especially in connection with the concept of "axial spondyloarthritis," it will be possible to include these patients in some of the previously mentioned categories. Probably the only case of AS without sacroiliitis quoted in the literature belongs here, despite the fact that the author states that this form occurs in 3 % of patients suffering from AS [23]. Two independent studies in families with HLA B27-positive probands with ankylosing spondylitis are of interest in this field. In the Cleveland study, 9 of 100 relatives of such probands ($n=30$) had typical clinical symptomatology of AS without corresponding X-ray changes on sacroiliac joints or the spine. In all nine subjects, a positive HLA B27 antigen (in contrast with asymptomatic relatives) was later confirmed. In the Leiden study of 101 relatives of 20 HLA B27 positive patients with AS, 13 of

86 relatives without sacroiliitis had inflammatory pain in the thoracic spine according to the Rome criteria for AS. Twelve of them were HLA B27 positive [24]. With regard to the fact that data on further development in these relatives are missing, it is not possible to rule out that it was a "pre-radiographic stage" of AS (group 1 in this case).

Conclusion: With the new concept of axial (and peripheral) spondyloarthritis, the diagnosis of "ankylosing spondylitis without sacroiliitis" will probably be extremely rare.

Acknowledgement This paper was supported by a research grant from the Ministry of Health of the Czech Republic No. 000 000 23728

References

1. Van der Linden SM, Valkenburg HA, Cats A (1984) Evaluation of the diagnostic criteria for ankylosing spondylitis: a proposal for modification of the New York criteria. Arthritis Rheum 27:361–368
2. Krebs W (1934) Das Roentgenbild des Beckensbei der Bechterewschen Krankheit. Fortschr Roentgenstrahlen 50:537–542
3. Moll JM, Haslock I, Macrae IF et al (1974) Associations between ankylosing spondylitis, psoriatic arthritis, Reiter's disease, the intestinal arthropathies and Behçet's syndrome. Medicine (Baltimore) 53:343–364
4. Amor B, Dougados M, Mijiyawa M (1990) Critères de classification des spondylarthropathies. Rev Rhum 57:85–89
5. Dougados M, van der Linden S, Juhlin R et al (1991) The European Spondylarthropathy Study Group preliminary criteria for the classification of spondylarthropathy. Arthritis Rheum 34:1218–1227
6. Kellgren JH, Jeffrey MR, Ball J (1963) The epidemiology of chronic rheumatism, vol I. Blackwell Scientific Publications, Oxford, pp 326–327
7. Bennett PH, Burch TA (1968) Population studies of the rheumatic diseases. Excerpta Medica Foundation, Amsterdam, pp 456–457
8. Mau W, Zeidler H, Mau R et al (1988) Clinical features and prognosis of patients with possible ankylosing spondylitis: results of a ten-year follow-up. J Rheumatol 15:1109–1114
9. Pavelka K et al (2007) Revmatologický ústav Praha. Abstrakta přednášek ze VII. Slapského symposia 12–26.V
10. Oostveen J, Prevo R, den Boer J et al (1999) Early detection of sacroiliitis on magnetic resonance imaging and subsequent development of sacroiliitis on plain radiography: a prospective, longitudinal study. J Rheumatol 26:1953–1958
11. Bennet AN, McGonagle D, O'Connor P et al (2008) Severity of baseline magnetic resonance imaging-evident sacroiliitis and HLA-B27 status in early inflammatory back pain predict radiographically evident ankylosing spondylitis at eight years. Arthritis Rheum 58:3413–3418
12. Rudwaleit M, Landewé R et al (2009) The development of Assessment of SpondyloArthritis International Society classification criteria for axial spondyloarthritis (part II): validation and final selection. Ann Rheum Dis 68:777–783
13. Rudwaleit M, Haibel H, Baraliakos X et al (2009) The early disease stage in axial spondylarthritis: results from the German Spondyloarthritis Inception Cohort. Arthritis Rheum 60:717–727
14. Chou CT, Lin KC, Wei JC et al (2005) Study of undifferentiated spondyloarthropathy among first-degree relatives of ankylosing spondylitis probands. Rheumatology (Oxford) 44:662–665

15. Brandt HC, Spiller I, Song IH et al (2007) Performance of referral recommendations in patients with chronic back pain and suspected axial spondyloarthritis. Ann Rheum Dis 66:1479–1484
16. Sieper J, Braun J, Rudwaleit M et al (2002) Ankylosing spondylitis: an overview. Ann Rheum Dis 61(Suppl3):iii8–iii18
17. Nagy SZ, Riler LE, Newby LG (1973) A social epidemiology of back pain in a general population. J Chronic Dis 26:769–779
18. Lee W, Reveille JD, Davis JC Jr et al (2007) Are there gender differences in severity of ankylosing spondylitis? Results from the PSOAS cohort. Ann Rheum Dis 66:633–638
19. Linder R, Hoffmann A, Brunner R (2004) Prevalence of the spondyloarthritidies in patients with uveitis. J Rheumatol 31:2226–2229
20. Balint PV, Kane D, Wilson H et al (2002) Ultrasonography of enthesial insertions in the lower limb in spondyloarthropathy. Ann Rheum Dis 61:905–910
21. Dekker-Saeys BJ, Meuwissen SG, Van-Der-Berg-Loonen EM (1978) Ankylosing spondylitis and inflammatory bowel disease II. Prevalence of peripheral arthritis, sacroiliitis and ankylosing spondylitis in patients suffering from inflammatory bowel disease. Ann Rheum Dis 37:33–35
22. Mader R (1999) Atypical clinical presentation of ankylosing spondylitis. Semin Arthritis Rheum 29(3):191–196
23. Pate D, Huslig EL (1985) Atypical presentation of ankylosing spondylitis: a case study. J Manipulative Physiol Ther 8(2):105–108
24. Khan MA, van der Linden SM, Kushner I et al (1985) Spondylitic disease without radiographic evidence of sacroiliitis in relatives of HLA B27 positive ankylosing spondylitis patients. Arthritis Rheum 28(1):40–43

Tophaceous Gout in the Spine Without Prior Hyperuricemia or Tophi in Other Locations

Jozef Rovenský and Jana Sedláková

Contents

Discussion 100
References 101

Abstract

The occurrence of gouty tophi is typical for the chronic stage of gouty arthritis. Tophaceous gout of the spine is rare. It is caused by the deposits of natrium urate crystals into the intervertebral space, intervertebral joints, and fibrous tissue, and it forms epidural masses. This paper presents an overview of published rare cases of sine syndrome in gout – evidence of tophi in the spine in patients previously not treated for gout – without prior documented hyperuricemia, arthritis attacks or tophi in other locations. In these cases, where there is no history of chronic gouty arthritis in a patient with back pain and neurological symptoms, diagnosis is difficult. Computed tomography and magnetic resonance imaging are helpful in the diagnosis, but a definitive diagnosis was established by the histopathological analysis of the material obtained by decompressive laminectomy or needle biopsy.

Gout is a clinical syndrome that occurs in people with hyperuricemia and is an inflammatory response of the body to the presence of natrium urate crystals. In its

J. Rovenský (✉)
National Institute of Rheumatic Diseases, Piešťany, Slovakia

Institute of Physiotherapy, Balneology and Therapeutic Rehabilitation, University of Saint Cyril and Methodius, Trnava, Piešťany, Slovakia
e-mail: jozef.rovensky@nurch.sk

J. Sedláková
National Institute of Rheumatic Diseases, Nábrežie I. Krasku 4, Piešťany 921 12, Slovakia

J. Rovensky et al. (eds.), *Sine Syndromes in Rheumatology*,
DOI 10.1007/978-3-7091-1541-1_14, © Springer-Verlag Wien 2014

natural course it goes through four clinical stages: (1) asymptomatic hyperuricemia, (2) acute attack, (3) intercritical gout, and (4) chronic gout.

The chronic stage of gouty arthritis is defined by the presence of tophi containing deposits of natrium urate. Tophi can be divided into bone tophi and soft tissue tophi. Typical localizations of soft tissue tophi are the ear lobe, first metatarsophalangeal (MTP1) joint of the foot, along the ulnar edge of the forearm, at the elbows (can cause dilation of olecranon bursae), over the extensor parts of the small joints of the hands, and at the Achilles tendon. They appear less frequently on eyelids, the tongue, in the cartilage of the airways, lungs, and rarely in the pericardium and heart valves.

In the tophi, secondary deposits of hydroxyapatite arise, which produce X-ray calcification-rich shadows. Tophi develop slowly and might not cause any problems for a long time. Sometimes they roll over the surface and drain chalky material. Tophi in the articular cartilage and subchondral bone give rise to chronic destructive arthropathy. Chronic tophaceous gout is associated with the development of secondary osteoarthritis which, along with polyarthritis and tophi, are involved in the development of severe, often bizarre deformities.

Spinal joints are not completely spared from urate deposition, but gouty spondylitis is very unusual. Spinal cord compression caused by tophi is considered rare [1].

In this review, we present the published cases of gout tophi in the spine as the first sign of tophaceous gout – without prior hyperuricemia, without symptoms of gouty arthritis or without the presence of tophi in other locations (Table 1).

Eight such cases were published since 1985. These were patients who sought medical assistance for acute or long-time progressive pain in the lumbar spine [2, 4–8]. Neurological examinations found signs of radiculopathy in the segments L4-S1 – numbness in the lower extremities. One patient had spasticity of the upper and lower extremities, reduced sensitivity to pain, and abnormal reflexes on the extremities. The patient had craniocervical transition affected by the disease [3].

No patient had a history of arthritis attacks or gout tophi in other locations. Medical history revealed hyperuricemia without treatment in only one patient, who had a kidney transplant 10 years before. A biopsy proved signs of chronic allograft rejection, and treatment included cyclosporin A and corticosteroids, all of which are risk factors for the development of gout [6]. At baseline, six patients had elevated levels of serum uric acid [2–6, 8], one had a normal level [5] and in one case, no uric acid values were reported [7].

In three cases, a suspicion was expressed for spondylodiscitis or epidural abscess, based on laboratory tests (elevated erythrocyte sedimentation rate, elevated C-reactive protein and leukocytes); the presence of erosions of covering surfaces of the vertebral bodies on x-ray increased the signal in the lumbar region on scintigraphy or imaging of soft tissue masses by MRI [4, 7, 8].

The material for histopathological diagnosis was obtained in five cases during the surgery – decompressive laminectomy and discectomy [2, 3, 5, 7, 8] and in three cases by percutaneous needle biopsy of the lesion point [4–6].

In one patient, swelling and joint pain of the first metatarsophalangeal joint of the left foot appeared during the postoperative course and colchicine was introduced

Table 1 Summary of published cases of tophi in the spine in patients without prior hyperuricemia or evidence of tophi in other locations

Published	Sex	Age	Symptoms	Gout, tophi in history	Uric acid µmol/l[a]	Sampling and location of material	Further findings/actions
1985 [2]	F	76	Radiculopathy	No	510	Decompressive laminectomy, L5	Edema and pain in left MTP1, colchicine
1987 [3]	M	69	Spasticity of limbs, abnormal reflex	No	500	Decompression, craniocervical border	
1988 [4]	M	44	Pain in lumbar spine	No	639	Percutaneous needle biopsy, L5-S1	NSAID, allopurinol
1995 [5]	M	61	Radiculopathy	No	395	Percutaneous needle biopsy, L4-5	Pain and edema in MTP1 10 years ago, without diagnosis/therapy
1995 [5]	F	71	Signs of radiculopathy	No	736	Decompressive laminectomy L4, discectomy L4-5	Additionally typical cysts and erosions of MTP1 on x-ray, therapy – allopurinol, colchicine
2000 [6]	M	27	Pain in lumbar spine	No tophi, hyperuricemia without treatment	710	Needle aspiration biopsy, L3-4	
2003 [7]	F	65	Radiculopathy, dysesthesia in dermatome L5-S1	No	Unknown	Decompressive laminectomy, L5-S1	Normal uric acid levels after surgery
2007 [8]	M	55	Radiculopathy	No	12.6 mg/dl (normal values 3–8.3)	Laminectomy L4, L4-5 discectomy	Normal uric acid levels after surgery, therapy – colchicine, NSAID

MTP1 first metatarsophalangeal joint, *NSAID* non-steroid anti-inflammatory drugs
[a]Normal values 100–400 µmol/l

into the therapy [2]. In another patient, after the evidence of tophi in the spine, an X-ray image of the feet was done, with typical cysts and erosions visible in the MTP1 joint [5]. One patient subsequently indicated three episodes of acute pain and swelling of the MTP1 joint 10 years ago, but without diagnosis and without treatment [5].

Discussion

In chronic gouty arthritis, tophi in the spine are rare. Overall, 46 such cases have been reported in the literature [8–12]. The compression of neural structures by a tophus is described mostly in patients with longstanding polyarticular tophaceous gout. If neurological symptoms occur in this group of patients, this option should be taken into consideration [13]. In our summary of published cases without history of gouty arthritis (Table 1), hyperuricemia or tophi in other locations, the diagnosis is more difficult at the onset of spinal pain and neurological symptoms.

Natrium urate crystals can be stored in the intervertebral space, in the intervertebral joints, in *ligamenta flava* and they can form an epidural mass. Described are cases with cervical, thoracic and lumbar spine crystals. In the cervical spine they can cause the destruction of the dens axis and atlanto-axial dislocation [13, 14], which resemble cervical spine involvement in rheumatoid arthritis. Gouty tophi can cause back pain and neurological symptoms of spinal cord compression or nerve roots compression – radiculopathy, myelopathy, and *cauda equina* syndrome [8].

Conventional radiographs of the spine show segment degeneration – intervertebral gap reduction, sclerotization of the covering surfaces of the vertebral bodies, spondylosis, and spondylolisthesis with spondylolysis, as well as defects and erosion of covering tabs [14], which may lead to a suspicion of spondylodiscitis. If computed tomography (CT) or magnetic resonance imaging (MRI) shows the presence of soft tissue masses, epidural abscess should also be considered in the differential diagnosis, especially if the patient has elevated levels of pro-inflammatory parameters [4, 7, 8].

The CT shows bone erosions, defects with sclerotic margins on covering surfaces of the vertebral bodies and in apophyseal joints that contain a hyperdense mass [15]. Gerster et al. [16] report that using computed tomography, the natrium urate deposits appear quite specifically as the masses with a density of 160 HU (Hounsfield units), which is slightly lower than the density of tophaceous masses with calcifications present (450 HU).

MRI displays tophus as a mass with intermediate to low homogeneous signal intensity on T1 weighted image, and heterogeneous intermediate to low signal intensity on T2 weighted image. After application of a contrast agent (CA), there is either a homogeneous saturation of the tophus or saturation of the peripheral ring (hypervascular granulation on the margin of tophi). The enhancement of CA in apophyseal joints is associated with hypervascular synovium [15–17].

In the group of patients described above (Table 1), despite the findings of diagnostic imaging methods that are not quite specific for the diagnosis, the definitive diagnosis has been made using the specimen obtained by decompressive laminectomy or puncture needle biopsy of the lesion of interest. During the differential diagnosis of spinal pain, neurological symptoms, CT and MRI-imaged soft tissue masses, one should think about the possibility of tophi in this area, especially in patients with longstanding chronic tophaceous gout.

References

1. Pavelka K (2000) Dna (Arthritis urica). In: Rovenský J, Pavelka K et al (eds) Klinická reumatológia. Osveta, Martin, pp 520–533
2. Varga J, Giampaolo C, Goldenberg DL (1985) Tophaceous gout of the spine in a patient with no peripheral tophi: case report and review of the literature. Arthritis Rheum 28:1312–1315
3. Van de Laar MA, Van Soesbergen RM, Matricali B (1987) Tophaceous gout of the cervical spine without peripheral tophi (letter). Arthritis Rheum 30:237–238
4. De Das S (1988) Intervertebral disc involvement in gout: brief report. J Bone Joint Surg Br 70-B:671
5. Fenton P, Young S, Prutis K (1995) Gout of the spine. Two case reports and review of the literature. J Bone Joint Surg Am 77-A:767–771
6. Thornton FJ, Torreggiani WC, Brennan P (2000) Tophaceus gout of the lumbar spine in a renal transplant patient: a case report and literature review. Eur J Radiol 36:123–125
7. Pao-Sheng Y, Jui-Feng L, Shin-Yuan C, Shiin-Zong L (2005) Tophaceous gout of the lumbar spine mimicking infectious spondylodiscitis and epidural abscess: MR imaging findings. J Clin Neurosci 12(1):44–46
8. Kyung-Soo S, Ki-Tack K, Sang-Hun L, Sung-Woo P, Yong-Koo P (2007) Tophaceous gout of the lumbar spine mimicking pyogenic discitis. Spine J 7:94–99
9. Nygaard HB, Shenoi S, Shukla S (2009) Lower back pain caused by tophaceous gout of the spine. Neurology 73:404
10. Ko K-H, Huang G-S, Chang W-C (2010) Tophaceous gout of the lumbar spine. J Clin Rheumatol 16(4):200
11. Yamamoto M, Tabeya T, Masaki Y et al (2012) Tophaceous gout in the cervical spine. Intern Med 51:325–328
12. Marinho F, Zeitoun-Eiss D, Renoux J, Brasseur J-L, Genestie C, Grenier P (2012) Tophaceous gout of the spine: case report and review of the literature. J Neuroradiol 39(2):123–126
13. Magid SK, Gray GE, Anand A (1981) Spinal cord compression by tophi in a patient with chronic polyarthritis: case report and literature review. Arthritis Rheum 24(11):1431–1434
14. Resnick D (1996) Gouthy arthritis. In: Resnick D (ed) Bone and joint imaging. W.B. Saunders Company, Philadelphia, pp 395–408
15. Souza AWS, Fontenele S, Carrete H Jr, Fernandes ARC, Ferrari AJL (2002) Involvement of the thoracic spine in tophaceous gout. A case report. Clin Exp Rheumatol 20:228–230
16. Gerster JC, Landry M, Dufresne L, Meuwly JZ (2002) Imaging of tophaceous gout: computed tomography provides specific images compared with magnetic resonance imaging and ultrasonography. Ann Rheum Dis 61:52–54
17. Hsu C-Z, Shih TT, Huang K-M, Chen P-Q, Sheu J-J, Li Z-W (2002) Tophaceous gout of the spine: MRI imaging features. Clin Radiol 57:919–925

Clinical and X-ray Findings of Sine Syndrome in Articular Chondrocalcinosis

Jozef Rovenský and Mária Krátka

Contents

Case Reports 108
Discussion 108
References 109
Bibliography 109

Abstract

Chondrocalcinosis is the disease caused by an abnormal accumulation of calcium pyrophosphate dihydrate crystals in the cartilage. The release of the crystals into the synovial space results in episodes of arthritis and secondary osteoarthritic changes. Chondrocalcinosis does not have a characteristic clinical presentation but rather typical radiological findings of calcifications of articular cartilages and ligaments. The pathognomonic sign is proof of calcium pyrophosphate dihydrate crystals with positive birefringence in polarized light.

Chondrocalcinosis affects knees, shoulders, hip joints and elbows most frequently. Small joints are affected only rarely. Involvement of the axial skeleton is even rarer and usually develops in more advanced stages of chondrocalcinosis. However, literary sources have also presented several interesting cases of sporadic spine involvement in patients without the peripheral joints being affected. Chondrocalcinosis can be a rare cause of common symptoms and we have the chance to reveal their correct etiology only if we have a high degree of suspicion.

J. Rovenský (✉)
National Institute of Rheumatic Diseases, Piešťany, Slovakia

Institute of Physiotherapy, Balneology and Therapeutic Rehabilitation, University of Saint Cyril and Methodius, Trnava, Piešťany, Slovakia
e-mail: jozef.rovensky@nurch.sk

M. Krátka
National Institute of Rheumatic Diseases, Nábrežie I. Krasku 4, Piešťany 921 12, Slovakia

J. Rovensky et al. (eds.), *Sine Syndromes in Rheumatology*,
DOI 10.1007/978-3-7091-1541-1_15, © Springer-Verlag Wien 2014

The first papers to present polyarticular chondrocalcinosis on the basis of characteristic skiagraphic findings were by Žitňan and Siťaj [1]. Kohn et al. [2] described, for the first time, calcium pyrophosphate dihydrate crystal deposition disease as "pseudogout syndrome," according to the finding of rhomboid microcrystals in synovial effusions. Chondrocalcinosis is caused by the inborn or acquired disorder of articular cartilages with the overproduction of inorganic pyrophosphate that results in its crystallization. Calcium pyrophosphate dihydrate crystals are deposited into collagen fibers of compromised areas of articular cartilages. Joint overload with the disruption of cartilage surface and subsequent release of crystals into synovial space leads to neutrophil and monocyte-macrophage fagocytosis, the release of inflammatory mediators and clinical manifestation of episodic arthritis affecting large joints more frequently due to their higher functional strain. The successive degradation of articular cartilages results in the development of secondary osteoarthritic and even destructive changes of the joints.

Clinical presentation of chondrocalcinosis is not characteristic. Typical signs of this disease include radiological proof of articular cartilage calcifications; however, the most important diagnostic method is the analysis of synovial effusion or bioptic material and finding of needle-shaped or rhomboid crystals of calcium pyrophosphate dihydrate in a optical microscope that look like anisotropic positive light-refracting formations.

The hereditary polyarticular type of chondrocalcinosis is characterized by early onset (as early as in the third decade); the arthropathy course is more progressive and is associated with marked inflammation. The sooner the first signs occur, the more serious and extensive they are. The sporadic oligoarticular type of chondrocalcinosis is characterized by later onset (fifth to seventh decade), changes that affect fibrous cartilages more often, and involvement is usually asymmetrical. The disease course is more stable, mild, latent and clinically harder to distinguish. Arthritic episodes are less severe and we usually observe only partial calcifications on X-rays.

The characteristic picture of calcifications on classical X-rays is caused by deposits of calcium pyrophosphate dihydrate that can be localized in intraarticular areas (fibrous and hyaline cartilages, synovium), paraarticular areas (articular capsule) and in extraarticular areas (tendons, especially at the place of their insertions, ligaments, bursae and soft fibrous tissue).

Calcifications have a chronic slow, but progressive course, and their distribution and extent are variable. They are continuous in the case of total calcifications; in partial calcifications they are less visible and intermittent. Cartilage involvement results in the development of secondary generalized arthrosis. The first osteoarthritic changes affect the weight-bearing joints and occur in the third to fifth decade, depending on functional loading and disease duration.

Fibrous cartilages (knee joint menisci, fibrous disc of the symphysis, and articular discs of radiocarpal joints) are most commonly affected. The calcification of fibrous cartilage is located inside it, and it is diffuse and has a mostly granular character on X-rays. Hyaline cartilage in large joints (knees, shoulders, hip joints and elbows) are less often affected, and cartilage in small joints (intercarpal, radiocarpal, talocrural, metacarpophalangeal, metatarsophalangeal, tarsal, sternoclavicular,

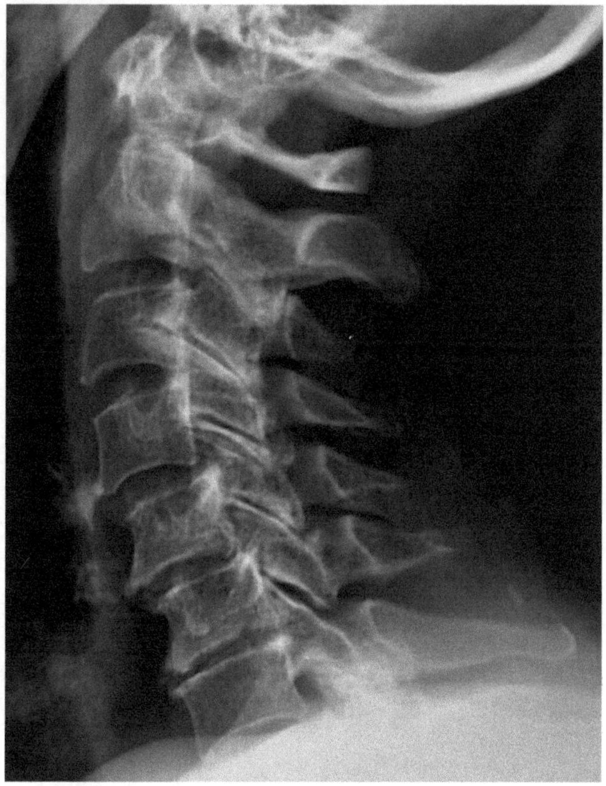

Fig. 1 X-ray picture of cervical spine affection

proximal and distal interphalangeal joints) are affected only rarely. Calcifications of hyaline cartilage are located in superficial layers heading to the synovial cavity, and they have a linear pattern on X-rays.

The involvement of the axial skeleton is even rarer. Calcifications of intervertebral discs are usually displayed in advanced stages of chondrocalcinosis. The spine can be involved in any part; the most frequently and markedly affected part is the cervical spine, with the lumbar spine involved less frequently and thoracic spine very rarely (Figs. 1, 2, and 3). The cause of the rare involvement of the spine in this disease is not known. Local tissue changes, e.g., previous injuries, surgical interventions, tissue necroses or degenerative disorders of the spine are considered to be predisposing factors.

A clinical manifestation of spine involvement in chondrocalcinosis varies, including cervical myelopathy, radiculopathy, spinal stenosis or *cauda equina* syndrome. The disease is often asymptomatic as well.

Involvement of the cervical segment is typically manifested as cervical myelopathy caused by crystal deposits in *ligamentum flavum* or atlanto-occipital ligament resulting in direct compression of the spinal cord or atlanto-axial subluxation. The involvement of the craniocervical junction can affect the exit points of cranial nerves with its subsequent neuropathy.

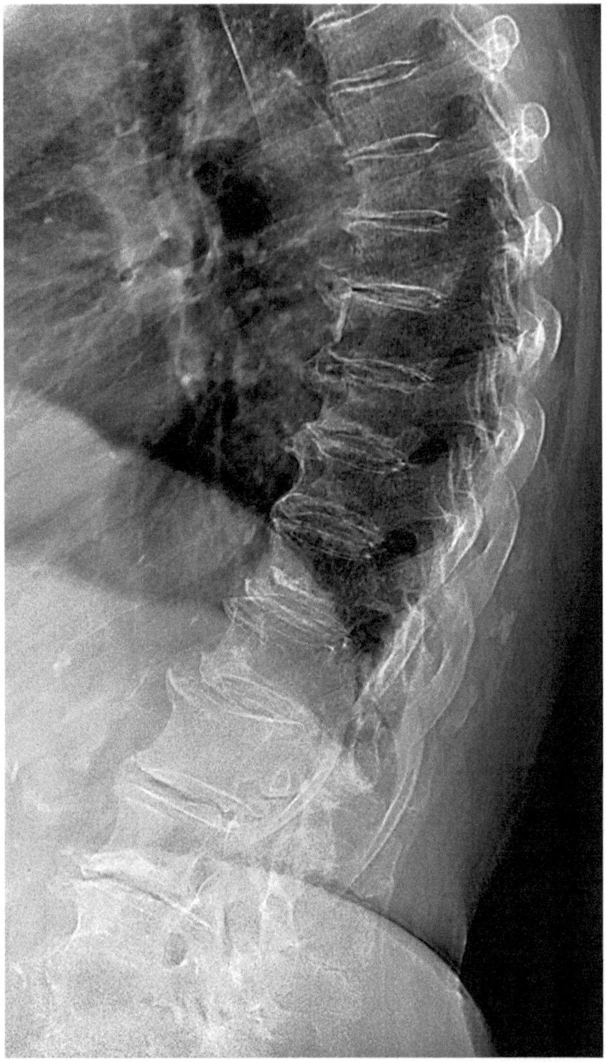

Fig. 2 X-ray picture of thoracic spine affection

In the lumbar part, crystals can be deposited into *ligamentum flavum*, intervertebral disc, joint capsule of intervertebral joints or into neuroforamina. *Cauda equina* syndrome occurs frequently. Spine affection can also have a lytic character causing pseudospondylolisthesis, or it can sporadically mimic spinal infection. Pre-operative diagnostics is complex and therefore the majority of patients are treated by surgical decompression and laminectomy. In the course of the surgery, chondrocalcinosis can be suspected if calcareous whitish material is found. The assumed diagnosis is subsequently confirmed by histological examination.

Deposits of pyrophosphate microcrystals in intervertebral discs form the picture of patchy or granular opacities mostly in the central part of intervertebral space and

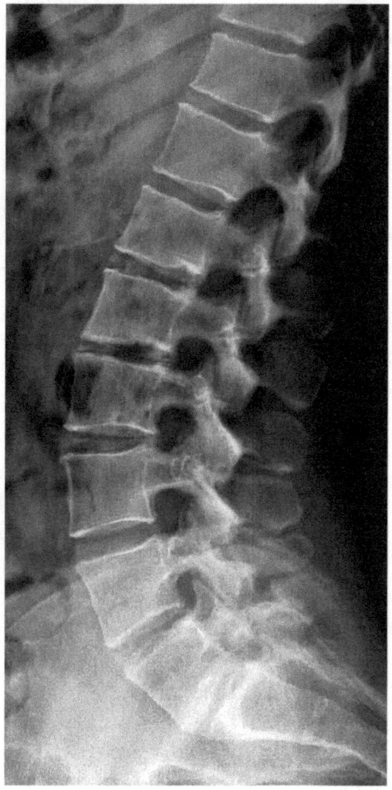

Fig. 3 X-ray picture of lumbar spine affection

at its ventral margin. The first discrete signs can be found on X-rays in the fourth decade, when the involvement of peripheral joints is usually fully developed. Opacities at the posterior margin of the spinal canal can also be displayed on X-rays. The straightening of cervical and lumbar lordosis and signs of early spondylosis, especially in affected lower segments, can be the accompanying signs. In the next 10 years, calcifications in intervertebral spaces become more intense, opacities become markedly granular or patchy and the structure in the ventral part gets denser. Sclerotization of the articular surface of the vertebral body becomes more pronounced, marginal osteophytes get bigger and the degeneration of affected discs with a subsequent narrowing of intervertebral spaces takes place along with disease progression.

CT scans show oval or nodular calcified lesions around the odontoid process of C2 vertebra or along the lamina of vertebral arches (usually lumbar) that can narrow the spinal canal. Oval or round, usually iso- or hypointense masses in *ligamentum flavum* resembling gout tophi, often hard to distinguish from hypointense signal of *ligamentum flavum* itself, can be displayed in T1- as well as T2-weighted MRI images. Deposits can also be found in interspinal and supraspinal ligaments, *ligamentum longitudinale posterius* and interspinal bursae. Although clinical symptoms, and especially characteristic radiological signs, can make the diagnosis of chondrocalcinosis very probable, the final diagnosis can be confirmed only by histological examination of material yielded from a biopsy or preoperative resection.

Case Reports

Literary sources also presented several interesting cases of sporadic involvement of cervical, lumbar and even of the thoracic spine in patients without having the peripheral joints affected.

An 86-year-old woman was admitted to the Clinic of Neurosurgery because of 6 months of weakness and stiffness of the upper as well as lower extremities. A CT scan of the cervical spine revealed larger hyperdense masses with multiple small calcifications localized at the C-1/2 level with apparent spinal cord compression. An MRI also showed signs of myelomalacia. Posterior decompression with the biopsy of epidural mass was subsequently indicated. The presence of calcium pyrophosphate crystals in an examined sample led to a final diagnosis: chondrocalcinosis causing compressive cervical myelopathy.

A 79-year-old woman was admitted to the Clinic of Neurosurgery with a history of progressive numbness of the lower extremities, worsening gait, repeated falls and a feeling of incomplete emptying of the bladder that lasted for 2 weeks. On the basis of clinical examination, X-ray findings of degenerative changes and MRI findings of *ligamentum flavum* hypertrophy with significant stenosis at the L-3/4 level, suspected spinal stenosis and *cauda equina* syndrome were confirmed. During the urgent laminectomy of the L-3 vertebra, calcareous material in the area of the *ligamentum flavum* was found. The ligament was inflamed, swollen and caused compression of the dural sac and nerve roots. A histological examination confirmed the presence of calcium pyrophosphate crystals and hence the final diagnosis: chondrocalcinosis.

A 72-year-old man was examined at the Clinic of Neurosurgery because of progressive pain in the left hemithorax for 6 months. The clinical examination was insignificant. An MRI showed a left-sided hernia of the Th9-10 disc with foraminal stenosis and compression of the Th10 nerve root. A mass adhering to the nerve root, probably a calcified epitheloid tumor, most likely a meningioma, was found during a left-sided Th9 hemilaminectomy. A subsequent histological examination of the sample in which rhomboid calcium pyrophosphate crystals with double refraction were found enabled the final diagnosis: chondrocalcinosis.

Discussion

Chondrocalcinosis affects the axial skeleton only rarely. The first signs of calcium pyrophosphate crystal deposits in characteristical areas of the spine are usually found in advanced stages of chondrocalcinosis. However, literary sources present sporadic cases of affection of cervical, lumbar and even of thoracic parts of the spine without the involvement of peripheral joints. Chondrocalcinois in the spine is often manifested by symptoms imitating much more common diseases. Therefore it is necessary to take into account this rare disease in differential diagnostics of vertebrogenic problems in patients and thus avoid unnecessary surgical procedures. The above-mentioned concept of the nosographic description of articular chondrocalcinosis comes under the picture of sine syndrome that has to be considered in clinical manifestation of this disease.

References

1. Žitňan D, Siťaj Š (1958) Multiple familial calcification of joint cartilage. Bratisl Lek Listy 28: 217–224
2. Kohn NN, Hughes RE, McCarty DJ Jr, Faires JS (1962) The significance of calcium phosphate crystals in the synovial fluid of arthritic patients: the "pseudogout syndrome". II. Identification of crystals. Ann Intern Med 56: 738–745

Bibliography

1. Lam HY, Cheung KY, Law SW, Fung KY (2007) Crystal arthropathy of the lumbar spine: a report of 4 cases. J Orthop Surg 15(1):94–101
2. McCarty DJ (1966) Pseudogout; articular chondrocalcinosis, calcium pyrophosphate crystal deposition disease. In: Hollander JL (ed) Arthritis and allied conditions. Lea and Febiger, Philadelphia, p 959
3. Molloy ES, McCarthy GM (2006) Calcium crystal deposition diseases: update on pathogenesis and manifestations. Rheum Dis Clin North Am 32:383–400
4. Resnick D (1989) Bone and joint imaging. W.B. Saunders Company, Philadelphia, pp 477–496
5. Rovenský J (2000) Klinická reumatológia. Osveta, Martin, p 167, 538
6. Srinivasan A, Belanger E, Woulfe J, Goyal M (2005) Calcium pyrophosphate dihydrate deposition disease resulting in cervical myelopathy. Can J Neurol Sci 32:109–111
7. Srinivasan V, Kesler H, Johnson M, Dorfman H, Walter K (2012) Tophaceous pseudogout of the thoracic spine. Acta Neurochir 154:747–750
8. Žitňan D (1985) Chondrocalcinosis articularis. Osveta, Martin, pp 42–56
9. Žitňan D, Siťaj Š (1963) Chondrocalcinosis articularis. Section I. Clinical and radiological study. Ann Rheum 22:144–167
10. Žlnay D, Žitňan D, Schultz P, Killingerová E (1993) Development of peculiar cartilage and tendinous changes in advanced hereditary articular chondrocalcinosis. Acta Rheumatol 11:47–54

Marfan Syndrome Sine Syndromes

Manfred Herold

Contents

Case Report No. 1 112
Case Report No. 2 113
Case Report No. 3 113
Case Report No. 4 113
Case Report No. 5 114
Conclusion 114
References 114

Abstract

Marfan syndrome (MFS) is a rare autosomal dominant connective tissue disorder that can affect many organ systems of the body. MFS is inherited as a dominant trait carried by the FBN1 gene, which encodes the connective protein fibrillin-1 [5]. The diagnosis is based on internationally defined classification criteria [9]. The majority of clinical manifestations of MFS increase with age, and diagnosis in early childhood may be difficult [6]. A follow-up monitoring in case of clinical suspicion of MFS is mandatory to initiate therapeutical interventions in time.

Marfan syndrome (MFS) is rare, but one of the most common inherited connective tissue disorders. The reported incidence is 1 in 5,000 [3, 10], the estimated prevalence 1 in 10,000–20,000 [14]. A family history of MFS has been found in 49 % of families with MFS individuals [13]. In about 25 % of the patients, the disorder arises from *de novo* mutations and occurs without a positive family history [3, 4].

M. Herold, MD, PhD
Rheumatology Unit, Department of Internal Medicine VI, Innsbruck Medical University, Anichstrasse 35, A-6020 Innsbruck, Tirol, Austria
e-mail: manfred.herold@i-med.ac.at

J. Rovensky et al. (eds.), *Sine Syndromes in Rheumatology*,
DOI 10.1007/978-3-7091-1541-1_16, © Springer-Verlag Wien 2014

People with MFS tend to be unusually tall, with long limbs and long, thin, slender, and spidery fingers and toes (so-called arachnodactyly). There is no geographic, ethnic or gender predisposition. MFS has a wide range of expressions, from mild to severe. The most serious complications are defects of the heart valves and aorta. The aortic root and arch diameter is significantly greater in persons with a family history of MFS and life expectancy is shorter. The key cardiovascular life-limiting symptom is the development of an aneurysm or dissection of the thoracic aorta, especially in patients younger than 50 years of age. MFS may also affect the skeleton, eyes, lungs, and, less frequently, the dura and skin. The diagnosis of MFS is primarily based on clinical features [9] but within the revised Ghent criteria, genetic analysis for FBN1 mutation are also included [8]. Early diagnosis is necessary to prevent fatal complications. There is no curative treatment for MFS, but careful medical observation and symptom-oriented interventions resulted in a marked increase in life expectancy. The mean age of death was 32 in 1972 [11], 41 in 1993 and 61 in 1996 [12]. The management of patients with MFS includes blood pressure control, restrictions on physical activities, and treatment of cardiovascular disorders including aortic dilatation, aortic dissection and mitral valve prolapse. Pharmacological treatment includes ß-blockers to slow down dilatation of the ascending aorta and prevent aortic aneurism, echocardiographic monitoring every year until the aortic root diameter exceeds 45 mm and every 6 months thereafter until the aortic root dilatation predisposes towards aortic rupture or the aortic root diameter exceeds 55 mm, or the aortic root diameter grows to more than 2 mm per year. For unknown reasons, life expectancy of patients with MFS is significantly lower in men than in women. Early diagnosis and tight disease control is mandatory for normal life expectancy.

Case Report No. 1 [2]

A 23-year-old man was seen by a cardiologist who suspected Marfan syndrome on the basis of the clinical symptoms. At age 27 his aorta had dilated to the extent that prophylactic surgery was indicated. The surgery was successful but the patient was not provided with detailed information about his MFS. The patient's brother was an active sportsman (basketball). The men's mother had died of a heart defect at age 36. The brother suddenly died at age 29 after collapsing during a basketball game. The postmortem showed a dissecting aortic aneurism. The significance of the suspected diagnosis of MFS given years before now became clear to the whole family as well as to the general practitioner. The medical care was optimal for the brother with MFS but not for the whole family, who should have been informed of the hereditary character of MFS.

Conclusion: If MFS is suspected, all relatives should be informed and evaluated for its signs and symptoms. If positive, prophylactic treatment to avoid MFS complications should be started immediately.

Case Report No. 2 [1]

A 19-year-old woman was first seen in an outpatient orthopedic department presenting with scoliosis of the thoracolumbar spine. X-rays showed a scoliosis of 60° left-convex with an apex at the first and second lumbar body. There were no signs of neurologic symptoms. A CT scan showed a progressive deformation of the thoraco-lumbar vertebrae with loss of normal vertebral concavity associated with progressive antero-lateral growth reduction and exaggeration of vertebral flattening associated with the development of marginal osteophytes which are suggestive for spinal osteoarthritis. The fundamental disease was Marfan syndrome.

Conclusion: Scoliosis affects about 60 % of MFS patients. In adult MFS, back pain caused by scoliosis is three times more frequent than in the general population. Ligamentous laxity is also a cause for precocious spinal osteoarthritis (OA) in MFS. Patients with spine deformities, joint hypermobility or early OA MFS as an underlying disease should be considered.

Case Report No. 3 [4]

A 50-year-old man with a history of smoking had severe chronic obstructive pulmonary disease and pulmonary hypertension. He has had spontaneous left (>20 years ago) and right (few months ago) pneumothoraces complicated by a persistent right-sided bronchopulmonary fistula. During the workup for lung transplantation the patient was diagnosed as having Marfan syndrome (MFS). Also a chronic superior mesenteric artery dissection was found.

Conclusion: Although pulmonary symptoms are not generally considered to be a main feature of MFS, many patients have some degree of underlying pulmonary pathology. Spontaneous pneumothorax is the most often described pathological feature. Lung histology shows distal acinar emphysema. These pathological findings are just beneath the pleural surface with sparing of the surrounding acini.

Case Report No. 4 [10]

A healthy 39-year-old man came to the university hospital complaining of a dry cough and progressive shortness of breath for 5 days. His shortness of breath was manifesting as orthopnea and paroxysmal nocturnal dyspnea, which he experienced these problems for the first time in his life; up until then he had no history of cardiac or respiratory disease and no history of prior hospitalizations. But there was a remarkable family history: his four brothers had all died of unknown reasons before reaching their first birthdays, and his mother had died suddenly at age 25.

An echocardiogram was performed and showed a severely dilated left ventricle, severe aortic regurgitation, a dilated aortic root and an ascending aorta (82 mm) with dissection extending from the root to the ascending aorta. Contrast-enhanced computed tomography of the chest revealed a large aneurysm of the ascending aorta measuring 9.9×9.0 cm with dissection. After successful surgery with graft replacement of the aortic valve, aortic root and ascending aorta with reimplantation of the coronary arteries into the graft, the patient recovered within few days.

Following surgery, the patient was examined by the ophtalmologist who found myopia but no signs of ectopialentis or any other ocular features of MFS. Screening of other family members was arranged and two of his children (ages 4 and 5) were found to have Marfanoid features with aortic root dilatation.

Conclusion: MFS should be recognized early, as medical and surgical management can avoid serious complications and improve life expectancy.

Case Report No. 5 [7]

A 47-year-old woman presented with a 5-year history of intermittent episodes of excruciating back pain confined to the sacral area. There was no radiation of pain, but the right leg occasionally "gave way," The back pain usually resolved spontaneously with rest. Recently she complained of urinary incontinence. Physical examination showed joint laxity and bilateral iridodonesis. During the course of her work-up with magnetic resonance imaging, extensive duralectasia was seen, beginning at level L5-S1 with expansion of the dura and thinning of the adjacent sacrum. There was a mild scalloping of the posterior lumbar vertebral bodies. Echocardiography revealed an increased diameter of the aortic root indicating MFS as underlying disease.

Conclusion: In patients with MFS of any age who have low back pain, radicular pain in the buttocks or legs, leg weakness or urinary incontinence, dural ectasia might be considered. Dural ectasia is a dilatation of the dural sac and may be seen as a major diagnostic criterion of MFS since it is rare in the general population.

Conclusion

Marfan syndrome is a rare hereditary connective tissue disorder that might affect various parts of the body. Symptoms may vary from mild to severe, and diagnosis, which is primarily based on clinical signs, may be difficult. Once diagnosed, prophylactic strategies such as blood pressure control, restriction of physical activities, echocardiography monitoring and beta blockers, can avoid life-limiting complications.

References

1. Al Kaissi A, Zwettler E, Ganger R, Schreiner S, Klaushofer K, Grill F (2013) Musculo-skeletal abnormalities in patients with Marfan syndrome. Clin Med Insights Arthritis Musculoskelet Disord 6:1–9

2. Arslan-Kirchner M, von Kodolitsch Y, Schmidtke J (2008) The importance of genetic testing in the clinical management of patients with Marfan syndrome and related disorders. Dtsch Arztebl Int 105:483–491
3. Collod-Béroud G, Boileau C (2002) Marfan syndrome in the third millennium. Eur J Hum Genet 10:673–681
4. Dyhdalo K, Farver C (2011) Pulmonary histologic changes in Marfan syndrome: a case series and literature review. Am J Clin Pathol 136(6):857–863
5. Faivre L, Collod-Beroud G, Child A, Callewaert B, Loeys BL, Binquet C, Gautier E, Arbustini E, Mayer K, Arslan-Kirchner M, Stheneur C, Kiotsekoglou A, Comeglio P, Marziliano N, Halliday D, Beroud C, Bonithon-Kopp C, Claustres M, Plauchu H, Robinson PN, Adès L, De Backer J, Coucke P, Francke U, De Paepe A, Boileau C, Jondeau G (2008) Contribution of molecular analyses in diagnosing Marfan syndrome and type I fibrillinopathies: an international study of 1009 probands. J Med Genet 45:384–390
6. Faivre L, Masurel-Paulet A, Collod-Béroud G, Callewaert BL, Child AH, Stheneur C, Binquet C, Gautier E, Chevallier B, Huet F, Loeys BL, Arbustini E, Mayer K, Arslan-Kirchner M, Kiotsekoglou A, Comeglio P, Grasso M, Halliday DJ, Béroud C, Bonithon-Kopp C, Claustres M, Robinson PN, Adès L, De Backer J, Coucke P, Francke U, De Paepe A, Boileau C, Jondeau G (2009) Clinical and molecular study of 320 children with Marfan syndrome and related type I fibrillinopathies in a series of 1009 probands with pathogenic FBN1 mutations. Pediatrics 123:391–398
7. Ho NC, Hadley DW, Jain PK, Francomano CA (2002) Case 47: duralectasia associated with Marfan syndrome. Radiology 223:767–771
8. Hoffjan S (2012) Genetic dissection of Marfan syndrome and related connective tissue disorders: an update 2012. Mol Syndromol 3:47–58
9. Loeys BL, Dietz HC, Braverman AC, Callewaert BL, De Backer J, Devereux RB, Hilhorst-Hofstee Y, Jondeau G, Faivre L, Milewicz DM, Pyeritz RE, Sponseller PD, Wordsworth P, De Paepe AM (2010) The revised Ghent nosology for the Marfan syndrome. J Med Genet 47:476–485
10. Samir N, Al-Fannah W, Theodorson T, Al-Mahrezi A (2012) Marfan syndrome: correct diagnosis can save lives. Sultan Qaboos Univ Med J 12:526–530
11. Silverman DI, Burton KJ, Gray J, Bosner MS, Kouchoukos NT, Roman MJ, Boxer M, Devereux RB, Tsipouras P (1995) Life expectancy in the Marfan syndrome. Am J Cardiol 15(75):157–160
12. Shapiri JR, Wright MJ (1999) The Marfan syndrome. http://cmbi.bjmu.edu.cn/uptodate/valvular%20and%20aortic%20disease/aorta/the%20marfan%20syndrome.htm
13. Yetman AT, Bornemeier RA, McCrindle BW (2003) Long-term outcome in patients with Marfan syndrome: is aortic dissection the only cause of sudden death? J Am Coll Cardiol 41:329–332
14. Yuan SM, Jing H (2010) Marfan's syndrome: an overview. Sao Paulo Med J 128:360–366

Index

A
Acute interstitial pneumonia
  chest HRCT scan, 6, 7
  corticosteroid therapy, 8
  decreased vital capacity, 7
  decreasing T-lymphocyte, 7
  ground glass opacities, chest X-ray, 6
  patient history, 5–6
  physical examination, 7
Amyopathic dermatomyositis
  acute interstitial pneumonia, 5–8
  cancer, 4
  cutaneous manifestation of, 2
  definition, 3–4
  diagnostic criteria, 2
  history of, 2–3
  interstitial pulmonary involvement, 4
  with juvenile onset, 3
  lupus erythematosus, 4
  magnetic resonance imaging, 3
  non-specific interstitial pneumonia, 45
  remission, 3
Ankylosing spondylitis
  atypical forms of, 93
  axial form, 92
  axial spondyloarthritis (AxSpA), 89
  descendent forms of, 92
  diagnosis of, 88
  ESSG criteria, 88
  MRI, 88–89
  Rome criteria, 94
  seronegative, 88
  undifferentiated, 88
  in women, 92
  X-ray manifestation, 88–89
Atypical forms of granulomatosis with polyangiitis (AF-GPA)
  c-ANCA positivity, 47
  clinical findings in, 46
  crescentic glomerulonephritis, 47
  mortality and morbidity of, 46, 47
  nodular form, 47
  overview of, 46
  secondary infection, 48
  with Sjögren's syndrome, 48
Axial spondyloarthritis (AxSpA), 89

B
Behcet' syndrome, 62

C
Cauda equina syndrome, 100, 105, 106, 108
Chondrocalcinosis
  calcium pyrophosphate dihydrate crystal deposition, 104
  case history, 108
  cauda equina syndrome, 106
  cervical spine affection, 105
  clinical presentation of, 104
  CT scans, 107–108
  fibrous cartilage calcification, 104–105
  hereditary polyarticular type, 104
  ligamentum flavum, 105
  lumbar spine affection, 105, 107
  polyarticular, 104
  thoracic spine affection, 105, 106

D
Dural ectasia, 114

G
Gouty arthritis. *See* Tophaceous gout
Granulomatosis with polyangiitis (GPA)
  clinical presentation, 52
  respiratory tract involvement
    bronchoscopy, 54
    case report, 56–57
    histopathological examination, 54–55

J. Rovensky et al. (eds.), *Sine Syndromes in Rheumatology*,
DOI 10.1007/978-3-7091-1541-1, © Springer-Verlag Wien 2014

Granulomatosis with polyangiitis (GPA) (*cont.*)
HRCT, 54
otorhinolaryngologic examination, 52
with pulmonary cavitations, 52, 53
serum c-ANCA antibodies detection, 52
skiagraphy/CT scan, 54
treatment and follow-up, 57–58
treatment of, 55–56
with ulcerous lesion, 52, 54

I

Idiopathic pulmonary fibrosis, UCTD
acid-base balance, 40
allergies, 40
bone densitometry, 41
bronchoalveolar lavage (BAL), 39
chest X-ray, 38, 40
diagnosis and treatment, 42
DLCO, 40
family history, 39
fibrobronchoscopy, 41
histopathological findings, 39
HRCT findings, 40, 41
past history, 39
physical examination, 40
present complaint, 40
social and working history, abuses, 40
spiroergometry, 40
spirometry, 40
transbronchial biopsy, 41–42
Idiopathic thrombocytopenic purpura, 14
Interstitial lung disease
chest HRCT scan, 26, 27
lung biopsy, 27
NSIP type, 27, 28
patient history, 26
physical examination, 26
Interstitial pulmonary involvement (IPI), 4, 5, 9

J

Juvenile idiopathic arthritis (JIA), 76

M

Marfan syndrome (MFS)
complications of, 112
diagnosis of, 112
dural ectasia, 114
incidence of, 111
management of, 112
pharmacological treatment, 112
pneumothorax, 113
prophylactic treatment, 112
scoliosis, 113
surgical management, 113–114

N

Necrotizing parotitis, 61–62
Non-specific interstitial pneumonia(NSIP) of the mixed type, 27–28

P

Pneumothorax, 113
Pretibial edema, 14
Psoriatic arthritis
clinical presentations and genetic aspects of, 83–84
inclusion criteria, 83
laboratory parameters, 82–83
oligoenthesoarthritic pattern, 84
past history, 82
present complaint, 82
undifferentiated spondylarthritis, 83

R

Rheumatoid arthritis
absence of erosive changes, X-rays
diagnostic summary, 67
laboratory parameters, 66
patient history, 66
X-ray findings, 66–67
ACR classification criteria, 71
DMARDs, 71–72
with dominating pulmonary involvement and oligosymptomatic articular involvement
after antibiotic administration, 69
bronchoscopic examination, 68–69
chest CT scan, 68
immunological laboratory parameters, 71
laboratory parameters, 68
patient history, 67
physical examination, 68
skiagraphy of, 69–70
lower doses administration, 71
RANKL antagonist, 72
rheumatic nodules, 72–73

S

Scoliosis, 113
Seronegative antiphospholipid syndrome (APS)
beta 2-glycoprotein I (beta 2 GPI) cofactor, 18
CAPS
aCL absence/decrease, 19
clinical presentation, 19
hemolytic-uremic syndrome, 19
multiorgan thrombotic-ischemic microvascular damage, 19
clinical signs, 17
definition, 18–19
elevated I-PAI level, 20
Seronegative catastrophic syndrome (CAPS), 19
aCL absence/decrease, 19
clinical presentation, 19
hemolytic-uremic syndrome, 19
multiorgan thrombotic-ischemic microvascular damage, 19
Sjögren's syndrome
with antimalarial drugs, 34
autoantibody profile in, 33
biochemical parameters, 32
bone marrow and trepanobiopsy examinations, 34
ENT examination, 33
immunoglobulin levels, 32
laboratory findings, 32
longitudinal follow-ups, 35
neck ultrasonography, 34
oncomarkers, 33
patient history, 32
salivary glands biopsy, 34
Schirmer's test positivity, 34
Still's disease
arthritis, 76
ILAR classification, 76
juvenile idiopathic arthritis (JIA), 76, 78–79
systemic form of juvenile idiopathic arthritis (sJIA), 76, 77
Systemic lupus erythematosus (SLE)
causes of negative results, 14–15
clinical sine syndromes in, 12
idiopathic thrombocytopenic purpura, 14
negative ANA antibodies, 12
pretibial edema, 14
renal biopsy, 13–14
skin manifestations, 12–13
Systemic sclerosis sine scleroderma
duration of, 25
finger infarctions, 24
with interstitial pulmonary involvement
chest HRCT scan, 26, 27
lung biopsy, 27
NSIP type, 27, 28
patient history, 26
physical examination, 26
mutilating form of, 25
PNAP III antibodies, 24
pulmonary involvement, 25
systemic lupus erythematosus, 25
undifferentiated connective tissue disease, 25–26
without skin involvement, 24
WPW syndrome, 25

T

Tophaceous gout
cauda equina syndrome, 100
classification, 98
conventional radiographs of, 100
CT, 100
histopathological diagnosis material, 98
hydroxyapatite deposits, 98
in other location, 98, 99
spondylodiscitis/epidural abscess, 98

U

Undifferentiated connective tissue disease (UCTD)
idiopathic pulmonary fibrosis
acid-base balance, 40
allergies, 40
bone densitometry, 41
bronchoalveolar lavage (BAL), 39
chest X-ray, 38, 40
diagnosis and treatment, 42
DLCO, 40
family history, 39
fibrobronchoscopy, 41
histopathological findings, 39
HRCT findings, 40, 41
past history, 39
physical examination, 40
present complaint, 40
social and working history, abuses, 40
spiroergometry, 40
spirometry, 40
transbronchial biopsy, 41–42

V
Vasculitis
Behcet' syndrome, 62
clinical manifestations, 60
GPA, 61
inflammation and coagulation, 60
necrotizing parotitis, 61–62
with venous thromboembolism (VTE), 61
Venous thromboembolism (VTE), 61

W
Wegener's granulomatosis. *See* Granulomatosis with polyangiitis (GPA)
Wissler-Fanconi syndrome, 76

FSC
www.fsc.org
MIX
Papier | Fördert gute Waldnutzung
FSC® C083411

Kolibri 360 GmbH
Ferdinand-Jühlke-Straße 7
99095 Erfurt, Deutschland
produktsicherheit@kolibri360.de